Growing Your Own Medicine

[2 in 1] Herbalism for Beginners Collection

Create Natural Remedies with Homegrown Medicinal Herbs for Holistic Healing and Sustainable Living

The Green Glow

Contents

An Introduction to Herbalism

How to Grow Your Own Medicine

Freebies For Our Supporters!

We've got a nice beginner recipe book for all of you herbal newbies out there. Just scan the code below to claim yours!

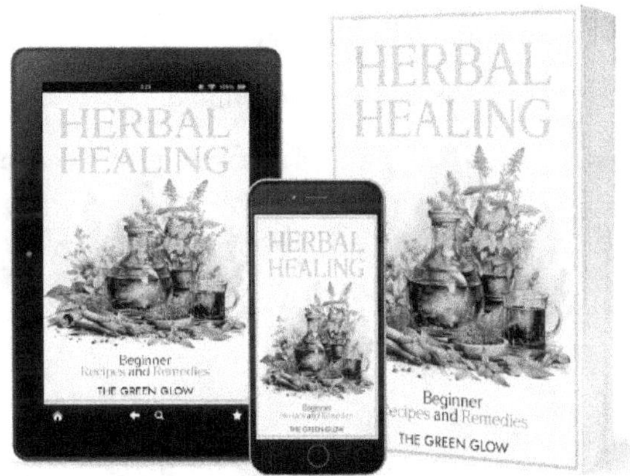

I want my freebie!

Join Our Budding Community!

We have a brand new community and we want **YOU** to help us grow! Are you willing to be one of the first seeds in our Facebook garden? Do you have any questions? Do you want share your herbal world with us and our glowing community? If you answered yes to any of these then, well, what are you waiting for? Just scan the code to join our community!

Join the Facebook group: Herbs, Heart, and Healing

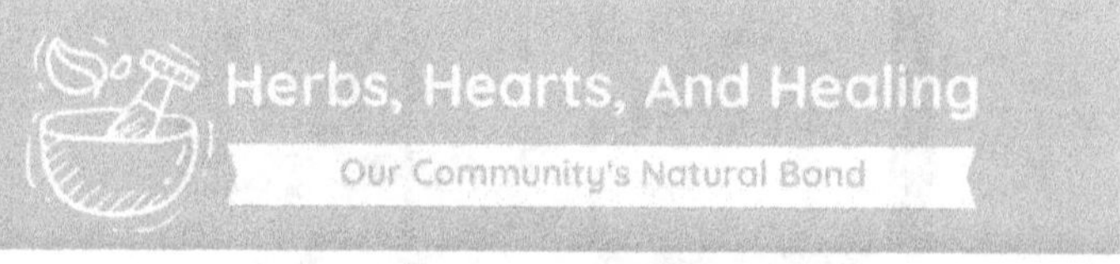

An Introduction to Herbalism

Step into Nature's Healing—From Growing Your Own Medicine to Crafting Herbal Teas for Vibrant Well-being

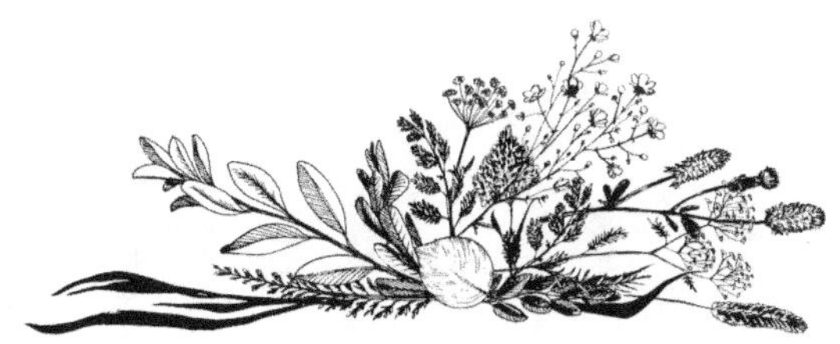

Introduction
The World of Herbalism

The greatest medicine of all is teaching people how not to need it.

— Hippocrates

Welcome, dear reader! Here, we start our engaging exploration into the fascinating world of herbalism. Are you ready? It's quite the journey. Who is this book for? You might be a seasoned herbalist looking to refresh your knowledge, a complete beginner keen to learn more, or someone looking to understand better what natural health is. Everyone is welcome here!

Today, herbal medicine is one of the most well-known examples of holistic health and natural remedies, combining age-old wisdom with innovative technology breakthroughs. The ancient practice is centered on using plant extracts for therapeutic purposes and transcends many cultures over time, reflecting our never-ending search for natural health remedies! To better understand herbalism, we need to look at the past, where it all started, how it can be used, and the complex relationship it shares with our more modern medical perspectives.

It's rather incredible how this ancient practice still remains so relevant today. But if we think about how our fast-paced modern world is scattered with synthetic medicines and other quick fixes, it's no wonder why so many individuals are opting to return to greener roots. We want a healthier way of caring for ourselves while keeping it as natural as possible, right? Plants possess the just healing powers we need!

So, with herbalism dating back to the start of human civilization, we glimpse its importance by looking at the ancient Egyptians, the Chinese, the indigenous people of America, and even European apothecaries during the Middle Ages... The list is endless, but luckily, we have a whole chapter dedicated to exploring the landscapes and cultures herbalism, also often referred to as traditional medicine, has touched. The wisdom has been passed down from generation to generation, including specific treatments and a way of looking at our health and well-being in general. The World Health Organization (WHO) explains traditional medicine is all the knowledge, skills, and practices that are based on native theories, beliefs, and experiences and are used in many cultures to keep individuals healthy and to prevent, diagnose, improve, or even treat various physical and mental illnesses (World Health Organization, 2019).

Something delicate lies between the respectful ways of doing things from the past and the harsh realities of modern pharmaceutical therapies. This bridge is made of more than just time.

It's also made of knowing and switching between how we view things. Our reliance on what is immediate, practical, and (often) synthetic has increased as our civilizations have progressed. We swapped hours of drying herbs in the sun for one minute at the drugstore checkout. But as we dig deeper, we start to see a theme that arises: a desire for authenticity. The story, which is as old as society itself, is not meant to downplay the progress made in modern medicine. Instead, it is intended to show how these discoveries can be used alongside ancient wisdom, where modern science and old herbal practices meet. Guess what? We have arrived! We are on the verge of rediscovering and redefining what health is.

As our story continues, we notice a significant change in how people think about their well-being these days. We soon realized that our modern medicines have some limitations alongside unwanted side effects. Think nausea, dizzy spells, and dry mouths (which is the least of our problems on that list).

It's become too easy to purchase that packet of pain pills and drink a few when we experience discomfort. It's like we revert to auto-pilot whenever we feel uncomfortable. Quick! What is the fastest way to feel at ease again? Think about it: We have a minor (or major) headache. What do we do? We immediately seek relief and reach for that medication. Did you ever stop to think whether there was a more natural way of getting rid of the pain? Because there is. The recent revival of herbalism can be linked to the increasing popularity of organic and natural lifestyles and a growing emphasis on wellness and one's own well-being. This comeback is not a passing trend but a more intentional shift toward person-centered, environmentally conscious, and body-honoring health solutions.

While herbalism has a long history, it has grown increasingly integrated with modern medicine in the twenty-first century. According to the National Centre for Complementary and Integrative Health (NCCIH), herbal supplements are critical to modern herbal medicine. These supplements complement one's diet and contain therapeutically useful herbs or botanicals (National Centre for Complementary and Integrative Health, 2023).

Herbalism has many applications but still has complicated legal and safety issues. For example, the Food and Drug Administration (FDA) in the United States establishes specific dietary supplement guidelines. These guidelines help us to draw attention to the regulatory and supervisory differences between prescription or over-the-counter drugs and nutritional supplements. Therefore, given that herbal medicines currently on the market cannot pass the stringent testing and standardization requirements for pharmaceuticals, herbalists and consumers (this is us) are urged to use our discretion and always be well-informed about the herbal products we purchase (National Centre for Complementary and Integrative Health, 2023). Something worth noting: It's always safer to consult your medical practitioner before making any changes to your diet or lifestyle, as we all respond differently to specific remedies. This includes the advice and guidance offered in this book.

It can be exciting to try something new, but we need to be cautious of the quantity and, most notably, the quality of our products. These dynamics make it more evident how relevant, trustworthy, and empirically based information is. Groups like the American Botanical Council (ABC) are leading this effort, which shares invaluable specifics on herbs and medicinal plants that have undergone in-depth analysis and evaluation by subject-matter experts. Their knowledge-sharing endeavors are intended to close the gap between conventional wisdom and modern science so that herbal treatments have a reliable foundation (American Botanical Council, 2023).

The ABC represents a more significant trend toward evidence-based herbalism, together with other groups of a similar kind. By integrating historical customs with cutting-edge scientific research, they aim to legitimize and enhance the use of herbs in medicine. This approach takes herbalism from mythology and stories to verified health research, which helps demystify the practice (especially for individuals starting). These organizations educate the public and medical professionals by emphasizing safety, effectiveness, and responsible use and support the idea that herbal medicines should become more widely accepted and integrated into traditional medical practice.

However, herbalism is much more than drinking tablets or liquids. It is a living, dynamic art that calls for a close relationship with the plant world and an innate understanding of the medicinal value that plants offer. Like in other contexts, such as kitchens, gardens, and natural settings, where people cultivate, harvest, and prepare plants in various ways, they engage with plants directly. Like the plants, the uses are diverse, from essential oils and beverages designed from therapeutic herbs to romantic and soothing herbal baths (and occasionally to spice up our latest dinner recipes). In addition to encouraging a greater degree of respect and a deeper connection with nature, this interactive aspect of herbalism educates us to take charge of our health, both inside and out.

Furthermore, the process of creating herbal medicines is person-centered. Herbal medicines can be customized to match your unique needs by considering factors such as your body, lifestyle, and pre-existing medical concerns, as opposed to the one-size-fits-all approach we see in conventional medicine. This individualization reflects a core principle of herbalism, which views healing and health as a personalized, holistic journey rather than just treating symptoms. You get to grow your medicine in the comfort of your home!

With all that said, herbalism has a bright future ahead of it, filled with possibilities and challenges as the twenty-first century progresses. Due to advancements in technology, more scientific support, and a growing focus on sustainable healthcare, herbal medicine will indeed become increasingly important in the future of world health. A well-balanced and thoughtful strategy for growing this practice is necessary since, at the same time, problems like quality control, ecological sustainability of plant resources, and the need for more widespread education and regulation continue.

Intending to enlighten, educate, and inspire you, this book embarks on an exciting journey throughout this extensive topic. These pages offer a thorough summary, practical tips, and a greater understanding of herbalism. This book will guide you on using herbs beyond fancy infused teas (we'll do that, too!). It's here to teach you precisely what herbalism is, how it has taken shape in the last few years (if not centuries), how you can successfully grow your own herb garden, and all the fascinating ways you can integrate herbs into your daily life. In our final chapter, we'll also explore how you can find your community of herbalists! Together, we'll appreciate the wisdom in herbs and plants as we flip each page and learn how to use their healing powers sustainably and ethically for our (and the planet's) well-being.

Chapter 1

The Rich Tapestry of Herbal History

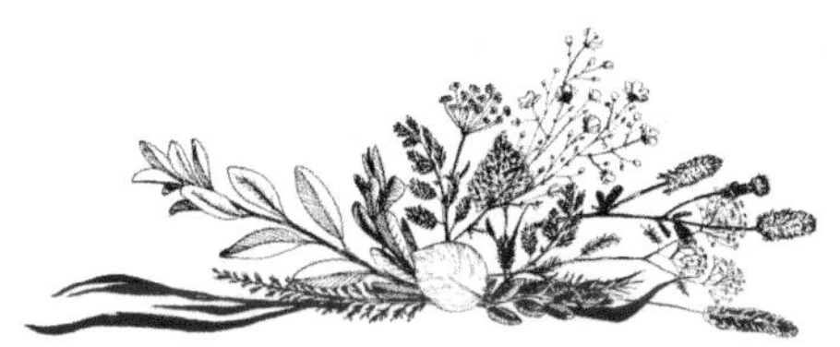

The art of healing comes from nature, not from the physician. Therefore the physician must start from nature, with an open mind.

— Paracelsus

Welcome to the unfolding narrative of herbal medicine. This journey is more than just an exploration of plants and their uses; it's an odyssey that spans millennia, encompassing cultural revolutions, deep-rooted wisdom, and, sometimes, radical shifts from conventional practices. The adventure we're on here isn't simply an intellectual stroll but a dynamic, informative adventure into how plants have shaped health and healing throughout different cultures.

The Origins of Herbal Medicine

Ancient Egyptian civilization, renowned for its tremendous architecture and complex hieroglyphs, was also extraordinarily progressive in its medical practices. Egyptian medicine uncovers a rich legacy that welcomed not only advanced surgical procedures and public health systems but also a philosophy that interconnected physical health with spiritual beliefs and the afterlife. Such a nuanced understanding of herbal remedies, blended seamlessly into everyday life, presents us with invaluable insights into the early chapters of herbal medicine.

The Ebers Papyrus and Beyond

Some 5,000 years ago, the bustling banks of the Nile were the cradle of not just architectural wonders but also of medical breakthroughs. The Ebers Papyrus, dating back to around 1500 B.C.E., is a pivotal witness to this era. It is one of the first complete medical records and contains just over 700 herbal prescriptions and treatments, revealing the Egyptians' extensive knowledge and use of medicinal plants. Ingredients such as aloe, garlic, juniper, and basil were used to address a spectrum of conditions, ranging from common digestive disorders to more complicated illnesses (Moorhouse, 2018; Pan et al., 2014; *The History of Herbal Medicine*, 2020). These are some of the very herbs we have in our kitchens today! Does anyone need a basil-infused remedy for an ancient touch of wellness?

Integration of Medicine and Religion

Have you ever thought about how our ancestors approached healing? It wasn't just about the physical symptoms. Take the ancient Egyptians, for instance. They didn't see medicine as we do today. For them, it was intertwined with their spiritual and religious beliefs. Textual evidence from both the Ebers Papyrus and the Edwin Smith Papyrus catalogs the variety of medicines and concoctions used but also outlines the accompanying chants and prayers. The merging of the physical and spiritual domains highlights an all-encompassing approach to treatment, where well-being is defined as a balance of body, mind, and spiritual harmony. How different would our modern healthcare be if we were treated with such a holistic approach?

Surgical Expertise and Public Health

Aside from their knowledge of herbal mixtures, the ancient Egyptians pioneered surgical treatments and public health advancements. They certainly exceeded our expectations. Surgical treatises like the Edwin Smith Papyrus reveal astonishingly advanced techniques, some of which remain impressive even by our modern standards. Moorhouse (2018) observes that the Egyptians' medical and surgical expertise was complemented by pioneering public health measures, including systems for water sanitation and waste disposal, evidencing a foresight in public health and hygiene far ahead of its era. Would ancient Egyptian surgeons be amazed or amused by our contemporary operating rooms?

Comparative Perspective and Legacy

Comparing the medical methodologies of the Egyptians with those of the next civilizations, like the Roman Empire, reveals both continuities and variations within the medical field. Egyptian medical thought was compelling, especially when it came to herbal medicine. They had foundational principles that later cultures embraced, modified, and advanced. It's incredible how their ideas influenced others. They valued their herbal practice, which went beyond traditional treatments. It was a system that brought together physical health, spiritual understanding, and community. Their sophisticated use of medicinal plants, combined with their advancements in surgical techniques and a well-organized public health structure, demonstrate a holistic view of medicine that is as captivating as it is instructional.

Neanderthals to Hippocrates: The Herbal Continuum

Did you know that our ancestors, even the Neanderthals, have been using medicinal plants for a long time? It's fascinating how profoundly rooted this practice is in our history. Archaeologists have discovered interesting evidence about Neanderthals, which includes remnants of yarrow, chamomile, and poplar at Neanderthal sites, suggesting that these early humans used different plants for medicinal reasons. It's fascinating to think about how people from over 60,000 years ago already had a natural understanding of how certain plants could heal. They knew that certain herbs had anti-inflammatory and pain-relieving properties. This discovery highlights the practical use of plants for health but also an early cognitive connection to nature and an early awareness of its potential to aid in healing and maintaining well-being (*The History of Herbal Medicine*, 2020).

The vast growth of herbal knowledge is signified in ancient Greece by the legendary physician Hippocrates, often called the "Father of Medicine." Hippocrates truly was ahead of his time! He believed in the power of observing natural causes and treatments for diseases, which was a significant change from the superstitious and mystical explanations that were widespread back then. He also had the innate knowledge that herbs can heal. One of his favorites was Willow bark, a remarkable salicylic acid compound, which is similar to the main ingredient in aspirin that we use today. His philosophy on healthcare can be witnessed through one of his very own sayings, "Let food be thy medicine, and medicine be thy food." This illustrates how important he believed our diet and natural remedies were for staying healthy. This enduring wisdom shows us how herbal medicine has been essential in healthcare for quite some time. It also shows how the medical field has changed and still affects our healthcare practices today. Some of Hippocrates' principles have laid the groundwork for a more holistic and balanced approach to health, integrating the natural healing power of herbs, and continue to resonate and inform modern herbal medicine and dietary practices (*The History of Herbal Medicine*, 2020).

Herbal Traditions Around the World

The practice of herbalism, essential to traditional medicine around the globe, uses around 350,000 different plant species. Beyond historical attraction, there is a modern return to this innate plant knowledge. It is recognized for its effectiveness, having minimal side effects, and its critical role in preventing microbial resistance to synthetic medications. This section will glimpse into some of the most significant and influential herbal traditions around the globe. Ancient texts, here we come.

Chinese Herbal Medicine

In China, the legendary emperor Shen Nong, often revered as the father of Chinese agriculture, is renowned for his monumental contributions to traditional Chinese medicine (TCM). Believed to have lived around 2500 B.C.E., Shen Nong is credited with tasting hundreds of herbs and identifying their medicinal properties, laying the foundation for using herbs in

Chinese healing practices. Much later, around 250 CE, these findings and teachings were methodically gathered in the ancient text *Shennong Ben Cao Jing*. This book is considered a cornerstone of traditional Chinese medicine because it organizes and discusses many plants and their medicinal characteristics and applications. It represents an enormous leap forward in herbal documentation and has played an instrumental role in shaping the course of Chinese herbal therapy, influencing not just China but also the broader Asian region (Pan et al., 2014). Because of its large and diverse geography, China is home to 31,000 plant species, which reflects its incredible biodiversity. Both indigenous and imported herbs are used in medicine because of these abundant natural resources and rich historical background. Today, China has a considerable effect on the global herbal industry, as evidenced by the approximately 8,000 Chinese herbal treatments sold to other countries.

The Indian Ayurvedic System

While Egypt and China were developing their medical systems, the Indian subcontinent wasn't far behind with its Ayurveda, dating back to around 3300 BCE. We're free to imagine a lifestyle where herbs are not just add-ons but essential elements of daily life. Ayurveda, literally the "science of life," is all about a balanced lifestyle–good food, yoga, meditation, and, of course, herbs. Their go-to guide is the "Charaka Samhita," attributed to the wise sage Charaka. Think of it as an ancient encyclopedia detailing thousands of plants and their uses in healing. This text doesn't only list remedies; it's about syncing your body, mind, and spirit for overall wellness. And guess what? The age-old wisdom in the "Charaka Samhita" isn't outdated; it's very much alive, influencing holistic health practices globally (Pan et al., 2014). Indian medicine is led by the philosophy that "everything can be a drug." They have about 45,000 plant species and 3,500 of those are for healing.

The European Chapter: Renaissance and Rebellion

During the Renaissance, Europe's herbal history took a turn. Influential works like Banckes's Herbal (1525) and Grete Herball (1526) emerged, shifting herbal wisdom into the mainstream. These books, written in the local tongues instead of elite Latin, brought herbs such as Rosemary and Chamomile into regular households, encouraging their use for day-to-day health and common ailments (*The History of Herbal Medicine*, 2020).

Nicholas Culpeper, an English botanist and herbalist, played a definitive role during this period. He was known for questioning established medical norms and focusing on distributing medical and herbal knowledge to the masses. His essential work, *The Complete Herbal*, published in 1653, was not in Latin but in straightforward English, making the subject of herbs that much more approachable and practical to the general public. Culpeper's comprehensive insights, combined with his personal experience, make "The Complete Herbal" a timeless resource in herbal medicine, appreciated for its real-world applications and because it's easy to understand (*The History of Herbal Medicine*, 2020).

Herbalism in the New World

As the Americas opened their doors to the world through colonization, the narrative of herbalism became a rich blend of indigenous, African, and European traditions. The herbal knowledge of Native Americans, especially, turned out to be a lifeline for European settlers. These indigenous populations brought various new therapeutic approaches and medicines, setting the stage for cultural interchange.

A noteworthy mention of the women in these cultures—their contributions during this historical era are particularly influential. Whether among indigenous communities or the new settlers, it was typically women who were responsible for the identification, collection, and preparation of medical herbs. This crucial responsibility placed them at the heart of health and wellness in their communities; their intimate knowledge of plant-based healing bridged gaps between cultures and ensured the well-being of their societies, highlighting an often-overlooked aspect of healthcare in these transformative times.

Modern Twists and Turns

The winding path herbalism has taken throughout the centuries has not always been as insightful and pleasant. Take the Salem Witch Trials in the 17th century, for instance. A misinterpretation and fear of herbal and natural healing practices partly fueled these infamous trials. As we flash forward to the early 20th century, we see the surprise of the pharmaceutical industry and a move toward uniform medical education. This shift placed herbalism on the back burner, often dismissing it as mere folklore rather than a legitimate medical practice (*The History of Herbal Medicine*, 2020).

But here is the plot twist: The last few decades have seen a vibrant renewal of interest in herbal medicine. This revival isn't just a whimsical throwback. It responds to the rising frustration with traditional healthcare and its potential risks. The crucial factor is that an abundance of scientific study is supporting many traditional medicines, increasing this newfound interest. Herbal medicine is getting back into the limelight, rejuvenated by new research findings, digital platforms spreading knowledge, and a worldwide community of passionate practitioners and advocates (Pan et al., 2014; *The History of Herbal Medicine*, 2020).

The Living Legacy

As we near the end of this chapter, it's clear that the story of herbal medicine isn't just a series of historical footnotes. It's a dynamic, ever-changing story with countless breakthroughs and much-needed insights. Our journey takes us from the historic Nile to today's state-of-the-art labs, with each effort adding another layer of understanding to how we view and use plants. At its heart, herbalism stays true to its grassroots origins —a body of knowledge lovingly nurtured and handed down through generations. By learning about and using the limitless possibilities of plants, we are making a conscious contribution to our future generations.

Chapter 2

Understanding Plant Power
Basics of Herbal Constituents

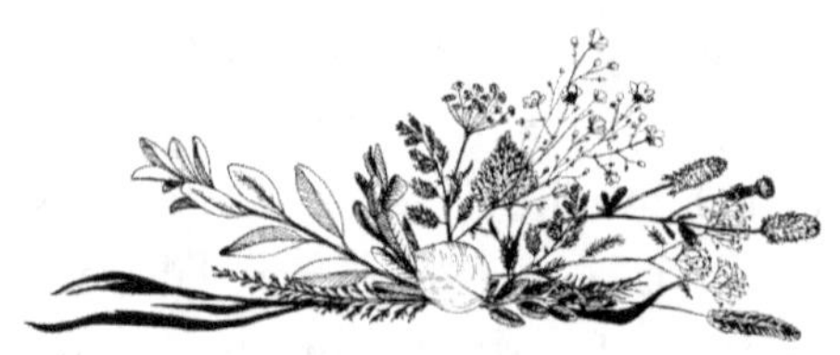

Plants are the young of the world, vessels of health and vigor; but they grope ever upward towards consciousness; the trees are imperfect men, and seem to bemoan their imprisonment, rooted in the ground.

— Ralph Waldo Emerson

Here, we venture into the basics of herbal constituents, discovering the incredible energy and complexity hidden within plants. This chapter highlights some key elements, such as flavonoids, tannins, terpenes, alkaloids, saponins, and phenolic acids. Each section will reveal how these natural components, often unnoticed, significantly contribute to a plant's life and, intriguingly, to our health and well-being.

Did you know that plants can influence everything from our mood and cognitive functions to our digestive, metabolic, and cardiovascular health? More importantly, we'll see how all these elements work together in synergy, which shows us just how interconnected nature truly is.

What Are Phytochemicals?

Strolling through a garden, have you ever considered you're amidst a vast, natural pharmacy? It's a space overflowing with nature's health-boosting agents: phytochemicals. These phytochemicals, nestled quietly within plants, are crucial both for plant vitality and our own health.

Let's explore phytochemicals through everyday experiences: The vibrant reds of tomatoes, the lush blues of berries, and the bright greens of leafy veggies, not to mention the inviting aroma of your morning herbal tea, are all the thanks to phytochemicals. They add a touch of much-needed color, enticing scents, and delicious flavors to our daily meals—can you imagine a world where you no longer taste or smell your favorite dish? Yet, phytochemicals go beyond our sensory pleasure; they are critical to our body's defense and count toward our health.

As we glimpse the spectrum of phytochemicals, we find flavonoids with their antioxidant prowess, protecting cells from aging and illness. Then there are tannins, offering bitter tastes in fruits and wines along with their protective qualities. The variety of phytochemicals is expansive, each contributing uniquely to our health and flavor.

Our meals are opportunities to embrace these tiny but mighty elements. By simply eating a crunchy apple, enjoying a cup of green tea, or adding cinnamon to oatmeal, you're tapping into a wealthy phytochemical source. Every piece of fruit, vegetable, and herb in our diet plays a significant part in our health.

The Green Glow

Could nature have always intended to nurture our health in such a harmonious way?

Flavonoids

You're enjoying a delicious pear or appreciating a warm cup of tea... Little do you realize that with every bite and sip, you're absorbing various beneficial compounds that champion our health—meet the flavonoids. These phytonutrients don't just splash color across our fruits and veggies; they are the hidden warriors in grains and our gardens.

Flavonoids are like nature's multi-functional toolkit, each meticulously designed to boost our health. Envision them as tiny yet effective protectors, arming our cells with antioxidant defenses, fending off free radicals, and building defensive walls against inflammation, viruses, and cancer (Santos & Silva, 2020). As you indulge in a plump berry or savor a glass of robust red wine, consider these microscopic soldiers diligently safeguarding our health, quietly working to revive our hearts and slow down the aging process.

The different types of flavonoids include:

- **Anthocyanins:** They provide our meals with vibrant reds, purples, and blues, as we can see in berries and grapes, adding not just color but also vitality.
- **Flavones:** Subtle yet significant, they can be found in various herbs and vegetables, also contributing to our wellness.

Furthermore, flavonoids are essential in ensuring our hearts beat consistently and healthily. Similarly, these compounds act as a gentle nudge to our brain cells, enhancing memory and cognitive functions—think of it as your morning coffee.

Tannins

We've all experienced the puckering sensation of an overly steeped tea or the dry mouthfeel after biting into an unripe persimmon. Tannins are responsible for that one-of-a-kind sensation! They make a bold statement wherever they happen to be. These phytochemicals are versatile protectors in the broader domain of plant chemistry and are much more than their bitter taste.

There are two types of tannins:

- **Hydrolyzable tannins:** These are found in oak galls and tea leaves.
- **Condensed tannins:** Commonly present in grapes, wine, and chocolate.

Tannins, often unnoticed, are vital in maintaining the intricate balance found in nature. Also, as a safeguard, they protect us against harmful microbes and viruses, creating challenging environments where these threats can't survive. Not only do they fend off potential pathogens, but they also serve as antioxidants, quietly guarding our cells against oxidative stress—a critical factor in aging and disease prevention (*American Herbal Pharmacopoeia*, 2023). Their antioxidant mastery ensures that our body's processes, including digestion and heart health, remain in excellent condition.

Now, let's connect some dots. The slight bitterness in your tea, perhaps your glass of red wine, or the durability of your leather jacket? That's tannins working their magic. They've enriched our history, being essential in traditional medicines for wound healing and inflammation, giving our food a unique edge, and even playing a crucial role in the leather industry. So, with tannins adding depth to both our palates and healthiness, it makes us wonder: What other plant-based wonders are subtly enhancing our daily lives?

Terpenes

Envision yourself entering a forest where the aromas of fresh pine, calming lavender, and energizing citrus zest mix harmoniously with each breath you take. That's what the terpenes are for; consider them nature's own fragrance experts! These aromatic compounds are actively involved in the field of health and well-being, along with offering us stunning scents in the air.

They take on roles like reducing inflammation, soothing pain, and fighting against bacterial and fungal adversaries. These compounds have tangible effects on our mood and stress levels, too! Consider the calmness that a lavender-scented bath offers after a long day or the refreshing sensation of peeling an orange —evidence of terpenes at work.

These small compounds in plants, such as sage, peppermint, and chamomile, go beyond their aromatic characteristics. They delve into complex health science areas, including their intriguing yet slightly evasive role in mediating estrogenic effects through alpha estrogen receptors (Canivenc-Lavier & Bennetau-Pelissero, 2023).

In both traditional and modern medicine, plants rich in these estrogen-mimicking terpenes are gaining more attention. More research is being done on its potential role in managing hormonal cancers, alleviating menopausal symptoms, and possibly influencing cardiovascular, immune, and inflammatory conditions. Terpenes in plants like clary sage, chamomile, and niaouli are often refined into concentrated essential oils, the very ones we use at home in our diffusers, to create a calming space while you go about your day.

Anethole, a standout in this group, found in fennel, star anise, and cumin, is notable for its traditional use in soothing digestion, easing premenstrual discomfort, and improving lactation. This illustrates how terpenes aren't just playing with our sense of smell; they're engaging in a kind of aromatic enchantment, weaving their magic into our health and daily lives. With their widespread influence, terpenes remind us there's always more to discover in the fascinating world of plant-based compounds.

Alkaloids

Alkaloids are the sharp-tongued members of the phytochemical family; much like tannins, they are often associated with a bitter taste. They are found in coffee, tea, and certain medicinal herbs; alkaloids such as caffeine, quinine, and morphine are renowned for their influential pharmacological effects. They've been used in medicine for their pain-relieving, anti-malaria, and stimulant properties. However, it's their dual nature– helpful in appropriate amounts and potentially harmful in excess– that reminds us of the importance of respecting and understanding natural compounds.

Saponins

Saponins may fly under the radar compared to other phytochemicals, but their roles are crucial and increasingly recognized. These compounds, famous for their soap-like foaminess in water, appear in our everyday eats like beans, quinoa, and ginseng. Saponins are more than simply nature's cleansers; they also have some highly effective health-promoting properties.

Their potential to improve immunity and lower cholesterol has drawn the attention of experts and health enthusiasts alike.

But that's just scratching the surface. These multitaskers are known for playing defense and protecting plants from pesky invaders like insects and microbes. What's more, these compounds are turning heads in the commercial world. Their unique combination of structural properties—a blend of a triterpene or steroid core with sugar chains—makes them notable not just in the health sphere but also in food, cosmetics, and pharmaceuticals.

Thanks to growing consumer interest in all things natural, along with their surfactant qualities—think natural soap—saponins are stepping into the spotlight in various industries. They're more than an unexplored ingredient; they represent a gateway to innovative applications. Yet, their complex nature presents challenges in processing ways to extract and purify them. Luckily, there is more research on the rise that not only sheds light on the sources and properties of saponins but also focuses on the nitty-gritty of their extraction, purification, and how processing impacts their structure and benefits. Saponins aren't just about making bubbles; they're emerging as dynamic participants searching for healthier, more natural product choices.

Phenolic Acids

Despite receiving less attention, phenolic acids are widely present in fruits, vegetables, grains, nuts, seeds, and nuts. They serve as fantastic antioxidants essential in preventing oxidative stress and related illnesses. Not only do they appear to have anti-inflammatory properties, but they may also help prevent long-term health issues, including diabetes and heart disease.

How Plants Affect the Human Body

The way plants interact with our bodies is truly incredible! It's like a magical embrace of complexity and effectiveness. As we know, aside from their nutritional significance, plant compounds can have a significant impact on our body's functioning, health, and overall well-being. But just how deep does it go? Let's have a look below.

Mood and Cognition

Just as a soothing cup of chamomile tea can calm our nerves, other remarkable herbs like Rhodiola rosea and ashwagandha have the ability to tweak our brain functions. These herbs contain adaptogens, which are the natural agents that help our bodies counter various stressors, whether physical, chemical, or biological. Rhodiola, well-known for its stress-buffering adaptogenic qualities, is essential in enhancing our mood and ensuring mental clarity and cognitive function. It regulates the body's stress responses, combats fatigue, and has been found effective in clinical trials for improving mood, reducing anxiety, and enhancing overall cognitive performance, especially under stress (Adaes, 2018; Güçlü-Üstündağ & Mazza, 2023).

Similarly, ashwagandha, another potent adaptogen, has shown impressive results in easing perimenopausal symptoms in women, significantly easing psychological, somatic-vegetative, and urogenital discomforts while positively affecting their hormonal balances (Gopal et al., 2021). This herbal duo underlines the potential of natural adaptogens to boost our mental well-being and cognitive resilience.

Digestive and Metabolic Health

Traditionally cherished herbs like peppermint, ginger, and fennel are known to relieve our stomach discomforts. But did you know these herbs and others like turmeric and cinnamon do more than just taste good? A recent study by Champagne et al. (2019) explored plant phytochemicals and their role in resistance against herbivores, suggesting potential health benefits for us, too. Phenolics, found in herbs like turmeric, show anti-inflammatory and antioxidant properties, which could be game-changers in tackling conditions like diabetes and obesity. Likewise, the terpenes in ginger and peppermint, which once defended plants against hungry critters, could be our best allies in digestive health. So next time you sprinkle some cinnamon or sip on peppermint tea, remember—Mother Nature is doing her thing without us having to try!

Cardiovascular Health

Flavonoid-rich plants, such as hawthorn and garlic, support cardiovascular well-being. They contribute to blood pressure modulation, help with lowering our cholesterol, and prevent our arteries from blockage. Similarly, herbs like green tea are a source of catechins, compounds Ruskovska et al. (2020) found to enhance blood circulation and decrease cholesterol levels. This study also revealed the subtle gene-regulatory effects of flavanols, such as those in green tea, highlighting their role in inflammation and lipid metabolism. The growing understanding of these molecular mechanisms can potentially guide us toward better-tailored nutritional advice in the future. In the meantime, enjoy your green tea!

The Harmony of Synergy in Plant-Based Compounds

In exploring the world of plant-based compounds, we're not just looking at individual elements but at how they work together to create effects far greater than the sum of their parts. Think of a plant as a complex puzzle. Each nutrient is a piece on its own impressive, but when combined, they create a stunning image that not only delights our senses but also helps boost our well-being.

Here are two examples of how nature collaborates to bring us the best of both worlds:

- **Green tea:** More than just a soothing drink, green tea is a prime example of synergy. Its catechins, or the powerful antioxidants, work with natural caffeine to provide a gentle, lasting energy uplift, contrasting the sharp kick we receive from our cup of coffee.
- **Turmeric and black pepper:** This duo is a synergy masterpiece. Curcumin in turmeric, enhanced by piperine in black pepper, increases curcumin's absorption, amplifying its joint anti-inflammatory properties. So, feel free to sprinkle it generously!

But how does this synergy work? Certain plant compound combinations can significantly boost our body's ability to absorb and use these nutrients. These phytochemicals address various health aspects or pathways, providing a broad and practical approach to help prevent and treat multiple conditions. It's like amplifying the health effects by knowing what works well together. In both traditional herbal medicine and age-old healing practices, the concept of synergy is vital.

So, if you want to add some of this magic to your own herbal practice, opt for whole plant extracts instead of isolated compounds that can capture the full range of a plant's healing abilities. Many health practitioners take years to customize their treatments; it takes time to develop precise and effective remedies, so be patient with yourself.

Grasping the concept of synergy in plants goes further than simply appreciating nature's complexity; it involves integrating this knowledge into how we manage our health. The collaboration among various plant compounds, such as antioxidants, vitamins, and minerals, represents a more unified approach to health, recognizing each component's vital role within a broader wellness context. As our understanding of plant chemistry expands, it can transform our health perspectives, directing us to align closer with the refined patterns found in nature. This philosophy isn't only intriguing; it's essential in redefining how we use our plants for health, highlighting the importance of seeing them as a holistic, interconnected network.

Chapter 3

Growing Your Own Green Pharmacy

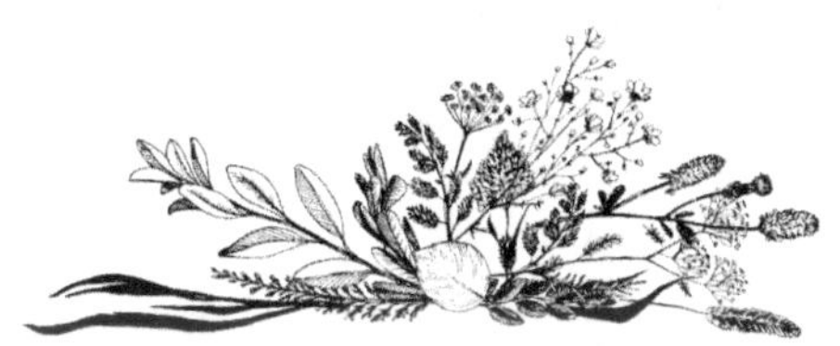

The love of gardening is a seed once sown that never dies.

— Gertrude Jekyll.

This is the chapter for cultivating green thumbs and nurturing curious minds! We can't deny the magic when we see a tiny seed grow into a lush green source of healing (plant power, am I right?). When we know how to grow our own herbs, it's about more than having fresh garnishing on hand for pasta night or to impress the dinner guests; it's about taking charge of our health and staying connected to nature.

So, get ready to set up your garden space, learn how to care for your herbs, which herbs you can quickly start off with, and a few more tips and tricks to help your plants thrive no matter the season. Let's get growing!

Setting Up Your Herb Garden

The joys of creating an herbal haven right in your backyard or on your windowsill! But first, we must ensure we choose the right space and use suitable soil. Here's how you know what is right for your garden (DeJohn, 2023):

Selecting the Right Spot

Essential factors to consider as you choose where to grow your plants:

- **Sunlight:** Most herbs enjoy full sun, which means they need at least 6–8 hours of sunlight daily. Keep an eye on your potential garden spots during the day to see which areas receive good sunlight. However, some herbs, like mint and parsley, like cool shaded spots.
- **Proximity to the house:** For ease, it's a good idea to place your garden near your kitchen or back door. This allows easy access when you need fresh herbs for cooking—think rosemary with the roast or fresh basil pesto paninis!
- **Drainage:** Make sure your space doesn't accumulate water after a rainy day. Herbs don't like "wet feet," meaning they don't thrive in waterlogged soil, so avoid forming mini ponds. Elevated beds or sloped areas usually provide better drainage.

Using the Right Soil

Some things to consider when it comes to the type of soil as you get ready to plant:

- **Soil types:** Herbs generally prefer well-draining soil with a pH level between 6.0 and 7.5. What would the ideal mix be? Loamy soil! It is a balanced mix of sand, silt, and clay. However, many herbs can tolerate various soil types if the water drains well.
- **Soil testing:** Before planting, consider testing your soil! There are many soil testing kits available at garden centers or online stores such as Amazon. It's a neat way to know your soil's secrets—like its pH and nutrient levels—and give your herbs precisely what they need.
- **Soil amendment:** Based on your soil test results, you might need to tweak your soil (*Rodale Institute*, 2021). For increasing drainage, you might consider adding organic compost or well-decomposed manure. To adjust the pH, you can use lime to raise the pH or sulfur to lower the pH.

City Garden Scapes

So, you might not have much backyard to grow your dream garden, and that's okay, too! Below are guidelines on how to grow a garden despite living in an urban area:

- **Limited space:** For those with space limitations, vertical gardening can be a game-changer. Use wall-mounted planters, one-of-a-kind hanging pots, or stylish trellises to maximize that vertical space.
- **Poor soil quality:** In urban areas, the existing soil might be degraded or of poor quality. Using raised beds with store-bought potting mix can create a more controlled environment for your herbs.

- **Balcony or window sills:** For apartment dwellers, balcony or windowsill gardens can be quite valuable! Always be sure to choose containers with good drainage and place them in areas that receive good sunlight, and you'll revel in green goodness in no time!

The main thing to take away from this section? Observe, adapt, and have fun along the way!

Basics of Planting, Nurturing, and Harvesting Medicinal Plants

So, you chose your spot, and you have the soil ready; now what? We plant, we nurture, and we harvest! Here is an essential step-by-step guide on how to take care of your new herb garden (Moss, 2023; *National Gardening Association*, 2023):

Planting

This seems obvious, but important nonetheless! Keep the following in mind as you plant your herbs:

- **Seeding:** Begin by selecting high-quality seeds from trusted sources. Some medicinal plants can also be propagated from cuttings or root divisions. Prepare a loose, well-draining soil mix, and plant the seeds or cuttings at the depth the plant prefers, as each species has a different liking.
- **Spacing:** Give them room to breathe! Ensure adequate spacing between plants to prevent overcrowding and stimulate air circulation, reducing the risk of fungal diseases.

Nurturing

Much like humans, our plants need some TLC, too. How can we show our plants love and care? By nurturing each species on their own terms. Below are all-around guidelines to consider:

- **Watering:** Medicinal plants, like all plants, need water, but the quantity and frequency will vary. Too much? They're flooded. Too little? They're parched. Over-watering can lead to root rot while under-watering can stress the plant. As a general rule, water them when the top inch of the soil feels dry. Aim for moist, not swampy.
- **Pruning:** Give your plants a slight trim now and then. By regularly pruning your plants, you encourage healthy growth! Remove any dead (droopy) or yellowing leaves and spent flowers. This not only improves their appearance but also redirects their energy to sprouting new growth.
- **Pest control:** Opt for organic pest control methods that are safe and eco-friendly. Natural options like neem oil, soapy solutions, and beneficial (plant-friendly) insects like ladybugs can help chase away common pests. Regularly check your plants for signs of uninvited critters and address these issues promptly.

Harvesting

Let's be honest; this is what we've all been waiting for: the harvest of our lush green growth! But let's not just take it greedily; we need to be mindful as we gather:

- **Leaves:** Have you ever wondered when to pluck those leaves? Right before the flower show begins! The best time to harvest leaves is just before the plant flowers when they have the highest concentration of active compounds. Cut leaves in the early morning as this is prime time, right after the dew has evaporated, but before the sun becomes too intense.
- **Roots:** Autumn is usually the best time to harvest roots, as the plant has stored energy in them throughout the summer. Gently unearth the plant, shake off the soil, and rinse the roots thoroughly.
- **Flowers:** Pick flowers as they open—hello, world! Again, early morning is optimal after the dew has dried before the midday sun. This ensures they keep their essential oils, contributing to their magical medicinal properties.
- **Maximizing potency:** To maintain the potency of the plant's harvested parts, dry them promptly. Spread them in a single layer on a suitable surface, such as a tray in a well-ventilated (breezy) area away from direct sunlight. Store dried materials in airtight containers, away from light and heat.
- **Shelf-life:** Properly dried and stored medicinal plant materials can last a year or more, but their potency decreases over time because, like fine wine, herbs age. It's a good idea to label containers with the date of harvest and use older stock first.

What a journey! The art of growing medicinal plants is filled with love and patience. Pay close attention to your planting, nurturing, and harvesting practices to ensure your plants offer the most therapeutic benefits. By being attentive and hands-on, you'll have a thriving green garden in no time—here's to your health and vitality!

Easy-to-Grow Herbs for Beginners

The world of herbs is expansive, and the list of species is simply overwhelming, especially for newer green thumbs, so below, you will discover a handful of beginner-friendly medicinal herbs (*Herbal Encyclopedia*, 2010; Neveln, 2016):

Mint (Mentha)

- **Cultivation needs:** Mint is a versatile plant, happy in partial shade and even in full sun. It thrives in well-draining soil and requires regular watering. Be cautious, as mint can be invasive; consider planting it in containers to keep it from taking over your garden.
- **Medicinal properties:** Mint is well-known for its digestive benefits. It can help soothe stomachaches, reduce gas, and is a natural remedy for nausea.
- **Home use:** Are you a regular tea drinker? Add mint! The leaves can also be added to salads, juices, or desserts for a minty flavor.

Basil (Ocimum basilicum)

- **Cultivation needs:** Basil loves full sun and thrives in moist, well-drained soil. Regularly pinch the stems to keep your plant full and delay flowering, giving flavorful leaves.
- **Medicinal properties:** While commonly recognized for its culinary uses, basil has anti-

inflammatory properties and benefits our digestive health.
- **Home use:** Known as the star ingredient in pesto, basil can be used in many dishes, bringing a fresh, aromatic flavor. Try different varieties for a twist—some offer hints of lemon, anise, or even cinnamon!

Lavender (Lavandula)

- **Cultivation needs:** Lavender needs full sun and well-draining, with slightly alkaline soil. It's drought-tolerant and doesn't like to be overwatered—don't drown them!
- **Medicinal properties:** Need to unwind and relax? Known for its relaxing and anxiety-reducing effects. It can also help alleviate headaches and improve sleep quality.
- **Home use:** Dried lavender buds can be added to sachets and placed in drawers or under your pillows to encourage relaxation. Lavender essential oils can be used for aromatherapy (a few essential oil drops in the diffuser ensure a restful night's sleep) or diluted for topical application.

Chives (Allium schoenoprasum)

- **Cultivation needs:** Chives also enjoy a spot with full sun to partial shade and prefer their soil moist and well-drained.
- **Medicinal properties:** Beyond their delicate onion flavor, chives are rich in vitamins and minerals, including vitamin K and manganese.

- **Home use:** Sprinkle them onto dishes for a mild, onion-like flavor. Guess what? Their pinkish-purple flowers are not only attractive but are also edible and can add beauty and taste to our salads!

Cilantro (*Coriandrum sativum*)

- **Cultivation needs:** This herb prefers cool weather, blooming as temperatures rise. Ensure it's planted in well-draining soil and gets plenty of sun.
- **Medicinal properties:** Cilantro is known to be rich in antioxidants and may help support our heart health.
- **Home use:** Widely used in Mexican and Asian cuisines, the fresh leaves bring a unique flavor. Some might find it unpalatable, while others can't get enough. Bonus? The seeds of this plant are known as coriander, a popular spice used in various dishes.

Fennel (*Foeniculum vulgare*)

- **Cultivation needs:** Fennel craves full sunlight and thrives in moist, well-drained soil.
- **Medicinal properties:** It has been used as a remedy for digestive issues, including heartburn, bloating, and loss of appetite.
- **Home use:** The nutty, anise-like flavor of fennel is welcomed into various dishes. And we can use the whole plant when cooking, as both its bulb and seeds are edible.

Lemon Balm (Melissa officinalis)

- **Cultivation needs:** Preferring a spot with either full sun or part shade, lemon balm flourishes in moist, well-draining soil.
- **Medicinal properties:** Lemon balm has a calming effect and can help relieve symptoms of anxiety or insomnia.
- **Home use:** Steep the fragrant leaves in hot water for a soothing herbal tea, or add them to dishes for a citrusy flavor; you might just pleasantly surprise your guests with a hint of citrus in your next salad.

Parsley (Petroselinum crispum)

- **Cultivation needs:** This easy-to-grow herb enjoys full sun to partial shade and moist, well-drained soil.
- **Medicinal properties:** Rich in vitamins, especially vitamin C, parsley is not just a garnish but a health booster! The more, the better.
- **Home use:** Add chopped parsley to elevate the flavors in your dishes, or use the curly variety to decorate your dinner plates.

Rosemary (Rosmarinus officinalis)

- **Cultivation needs:** Favoring full sunlight, rosemary needs well-draining soil and doesn't like to sit in water; do not overwater this variety.
- **Medicinal properties:** Known to improve our concentration, rosemary also has anti-inflammatory benefits.

- **Home use:** Their aromatic leaves are perfect for flavoring meats and vegetables. Try adding it to your bread dough; if you're feeling Greek, infuse your extra virgin olive oil with a sprig or two.

Thyme (Thymus vulgaris)

- **Cultivation needs:** Thyme loves full sun and prefers light, well-draining soil.
- **Medicinal properties:** This plant is known for its antibacterial properties and can help with respiratory issues—so you can just breathe.
- **Home use:** Infuse your dishes with the intense, earthy aroma of thyme, either fresh or dried. It pairs beautifully with meats and roasted vegetables.

Thus, in essence, these herbs are ideal for beginners like yourself and have a ton of health benefits. Enjoy the satisfaction of knowing that the medicinal plants you've worked so hard to nurture and develop are coming fresh from your own garden.

Seasonal Tips for Herb Cultivation

As with all things in life, herbs change with the seasons. Your question, then, is, how do you keep them thriving all year long? Let's have a look at what each season brings (Richter, 2023):

Spring

- **Planting:** As the last frost disappears, it's the ideal time to plant most herbs. Seeds or young plants can be introduced to well-prepared beds that have premium soil.

- **Fertilization:** Add a light, balanced fertilizer to help jump-start their growth after the more dormant winter months.
- **Pruning:** Spring is also the prime time for pruning. Cut back any dead stems from the previous year to make way for new, vibrant growth.

Summer

- **Watering:** Hydrate to keep them glowing and growing! The summer heat means your herbs will need more frequent watering. However, avoid over-watering, as you don't want them to be soggy.
- **Harvesting:** This is it! It's time to pick those stunning greens. Summer is the peak harvesting time for most herbs. Always harvest in the morning for the best flavor, and be sure you never take more than one-third of the plant; they need some leaves to keep doing their thing.

Autumn

- **Preparing for winter:** As cooler temperatures start rolling in, it's time to provide them with some snug, so consider putting mulch around your herbs to provide that insulation (Iannotti, 2022). If you have perennial herbs, trim them to encourage more vigorous growth in spring.
- **Transition them indoors:** If you live in an area with harsh winters, consider moving some of your herbs to pots and bringing them indoors. They'll appreciate the indoor warmth.

Winter

- **Indoor care:** Herbs inside need a sunny spot; your window should be perfect; remember to water them sparingly. Ensure good air circulation by opening a window for fresh air and to prevent mold from forming.
- **Protection:** For outdoor perennial herbs, provide extra love and keep them well-mulched. Some, like rosemary, may need more protection, like a burlap wrap in areas with severe frost.

General Tips for Changing Seasons

- **Indoor vs. outdoor:** If you're transferring plants indoors or out with the changing seasons, don't rush the process; rather, acclimate them gradually. Start by placing them in their new environment for a few hours each day, slowly increasing the time spent in their new space.
- **Weather watch:** Always watch the forecast, as Mother Nature can be unpredictable. A sudden frost or scorching day, in particular, heatwaves, can catch us off guard, so be ready with things like frost cloths or shade nets to keep your herbs thriving.

In this chapter, we've had the pleasure of looking into the incredible world of gardening and the many benefits it brings. From getting your space ready to the excitement of harvesting, every step teaches us the importance of patience, taking care, and appreciating our close connection with nature. As you start your gardening journey, take your time, learn as you go, and, most importantly, have fun along the way! Happy gardening to you!

Chapter 4

Herbal Teas

Sips of Wellness

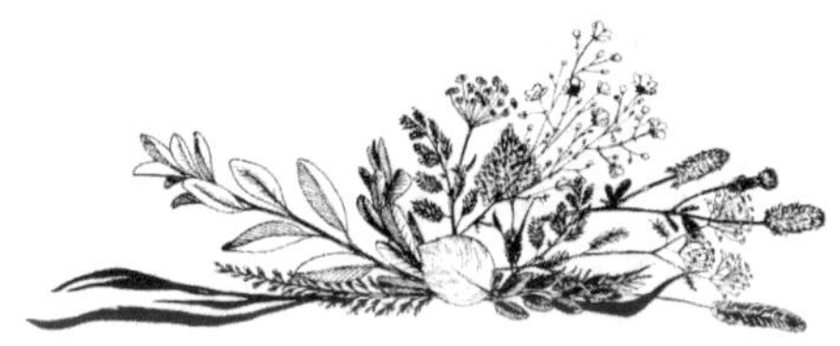

There is something in the nature of tea that leads us into a world of quiet contemplation of life.

— Lin Yutang

Welcome to the comfy corner of Chapter 4! Here, we'll explore the vibrant world of herbal brews—a wealth of vibrancy in every cup. With every leaf and root infused in hot water, a simple sip can be a source of healing joy and bring us closer to the wonders of nature.

We'll discover the benefits of herbal beverages outside the traditional tea leaf, turning every cup into a personal health remedy and a soothing ritual. We'll even make our herbal blends! Get ready to discover the world of herbal teas and how they can add to our daily dose of well-being.

The Essence of Herbal Teas

Discover the aromatic world of herbal teas and experience a legacy that is both ageless and wholesome (*The Herb Guide*, 2023). These are more than simply teas—consider the many combinations of leaves, flowers, seeds, and roots that give benefits beyond the flavor. Every cup connects us to a history of healers who have harnessed the life-sustaining power of plants, stretching from ancient cultures to modern health enthusiasts. Consider mint, which energizes; chamomile, which calms; and echinacea, which protects us like our own plant bodyguard!

Brewing the Perfect Cup: An Art and Science

Now, let's talk about crafting that perfect cup of herbal tea—a blend of intuition and precision, a gentle process where art and science meet right in your kitchen!

Here's how to make magic with your herbal teas (*TeaUSA*, 2013):

- **Water:** Begin with the most purified water; filtered or spring water is best. Tap water will do if it's not too alkaline.
- **Your chosen herb:** Place your chosen herbs in a teapot or infuser. Loose leaves prefer space to expand and release their full potential; they're quite the free spirits.
- **Temperature:** Each herb has its own favored temperature. Tender buds and petals like a soft heat, somewhere between 160 and 180 °F, while the hardy roots and barks are all about the heat and can endure up to 212 °F.

- **Timing is everything:** The steeping time sets the rhythm for your tea's flavor; a quick 3–5 minutes usually hits the mark, but if you're after a more full-bodied taste, feel free to steep up to 10 minutes.
- **Storage them safely:** To keep your herbs vibrant and compelling, store them in airtight containers away from light and warmth; a dark pantry or cupboard is perfect.

If you want to experiment, you are welcome to do so! The rules of brewing the perfect pot are not set in stone, so adjust the times and temperatures as you find what works for you.

Here is guidance on how to tailor your next brew:

- **Customize the strength:** Want a stronger sip? For a more robust flavor, add more herbs, but remember, steeping it for too long might make it bitter.
- **For the sweet tooth:** If you're after a touch of sweetness, honey or stevia are your go-to companions —they'll harmonize with your brew without overpowering it.
- **Fresh citrus:** A splash of lemon or orange peel can elevate the lighter notes of your tea and add some fresh summer tones!
- **Cold brew:** For those who favor a chilled sip, let your mixture mingle in cold water in the refrigerator overnight. It offers a gentle approach for a mellow taste.
- **Adding milk:** Milk or a dairy-free alternative can provide your tea with creamy luxury, perfect for

taming bolder infusions into a silky-smooth experience.

Remember, adventurous tea blenders, that each cup is your own custom-made elixir, and there is a certain amount of satisfaction in identifying the blend designed especially for you. Dare to combine flavor with ease, allowing each cup to honor both your creativity and respected tradition.

The Herbal Tea Pantry: Our Essentials for Wellness

Let's enter the herbal tea pantry, where delicious flavors and well-being go hand-in-hand. In the world of herbal teas, there are plenty! So here is a list with a few notable ones to know about (Jones, 2017; Wack, 2021):

- **Chamomile:** Think of chamomile as a gentle caress for your senses. With subtle floral hints and a soft golden hue, this herb is a lullaby in a cup, perfect for easing into a peaceful sleep.
- **Peppermint:** This one's the life of the party in the tea world, with its invigorating scent and a refreshing taste that wakes up our taste buds! It's a go-to for soothing an upset stomach.
- **Lavender:** A sip of lavender tea is like strolling through a field of purple flowers somewhere in the South of France! It's a calming source for those restless nights and a go-to for soothing stress.
- **Ginger:** Bold and spicy, ginger brings a warming zest perfect for digestion and energizing our senses! Simmer some freshly sliced ginger for a strong brew that ignites good health.

- **Echinacea:** Gentle floral notes with a touch of zest, echinacea is like a shield for our immune systems. Just a short infusion period is enough to prepare this fortifying drink.
- **Hibiscus:** Hibiscus blooms give your cup a ruby-red color and a tart flavor full of vitality and vitamins.
- **Rosehip:** Rich in vitamin C and friendly to your skin, the subtle, fruity charm of rosehip makes a rejuvenating tea that's beauty in a cup.
- **Nettle:** This underrated herb is a nutritional powerhouse, dense with minerals, and supports our overall health. Once simmered, it transforms into a deeply nourishing beverage.
- **Licorice root:** Naturally sweet and comforting, licorice root brings a smooth, soothing quality to any blend, perfect for calming a sore throat and easing anxiety.
- **Dandelion root:** Beyond its reputation as a stubborn weed, the dandelion's root is a detoxifying ally, supporting our liver function.
- **Tulsi (holy basil):** Sacred in many traditions, tulsi's unique flavor is at the heart of many restorative teas.
- **Cinnamon:** This familiar spice brings warmth and a hint of sweetness, promoting digestion and adding a cozy note to any tea blend.
- **Cardamom:** Fragrant and slightly spicy, cardamom pods infuse a distinctive, therapeutic flavor.
- **Butterfly pea flower:** With a vibrant blue hue, this tea is high in antioxidants and has anti-inflammatory and cognitive benefits.
- **Rooibos:** Grown in South African bushes, caffeine-

free rooibos is packed with antioxidants and is excellent for our heart health.

- **Lemongrass:** This citrusy herb balances digestive health, antimicrobial properties, and anxiety alleviation in a refreshing method.
- **Cota (Navajo tea):** An indigenous brew with earthy notes, Cota comforts the digestive system with its gentle touch.

Embrace these herbal heroes in your tea pantry, and you'll not only craft cups of comfort but also brew well-being into each day. Experiment with delight, sip with intent, and watch your wellness garden grow one cup at a time.

Creating Your Own Blends

This is the space where you can be creative. It's all about mixing and matching, finding the perfect matches in flavor and function (*American Herbalists Guild*, 2013):

- **Flavor fusion:** Each herb has a flavor profile—mint is cooling, cinnamon is warming, chamomile is soothing, and so on. Learning the basic profiles will serve as your guide to blending. You want to achieve a harmony where no herb overpowers the other unless that's what you want. Consider how the flavors will interact. Some flavors naturally click, such as mint and lemon, while others bring out the best in each other when paired, like rose and hibiscus, for example. Start with a foundation—mild green tea or the ever-versatile rooibos—then introduce a complementary note such as a zesty citrus or a sweet berry, and then a final touch for that extra tang, consider adding a sprinkle of cinnamon or a slice of ginger.

- **Combining for wellness:** Have you considered tailoring your tea to your wellness goals? Decide what the goal of your tea is. For relaxation, you might focus on herbs like lavender, chamomile, and lemon balm. For a digestive aid, peppermint, ginger, and fennel might be your go-to.

- **Getting the ratio right:** When creating a blend, a beginner-friendly method uses three parts of your base herb, one part of a complementary herb, and one of an accent herb. This isn't a strict rule but rather a starting point! The "base" is usually the dominant flavor or the herb with the preferred primary effect. The "complementary" adds depth and supports the primary function, while the "accent" introduces a contrasting note, often for a touch of complexity or a hint of sharpness to elevate the overall blend. Don't be afraid to try odd pairings! For example, a base of green tea might be enhanced with the floral notes of rose petals as a complement and a pinch of black pepper as an accent for an unexpected kick.

Here are recipes to get you started at home (*Simple Loose Leaf Tea Company*, 2020):

Lemon and Elderflower Tea

This blend is perfect for those looking to combat the symptoms of the common cold (goodbye sniffles)!

Blend the following for one cup:

- 1 tablespoon of elderflowers—fresh or dried

The Green Glow

- 1–2 teaspoons of lemon juice
- 1 teaspoon of honey

Classic Cinnamon and Apple Tea

A timeless herbal fruit tea blend that's incredibly cozy in cooler weather.

The following is enough for one cup:

- 1 tablespoon of dried apple pieces
- ½ tablespoon of crushed cinnamon bark

Chamomile and Lemon Balm Sleep Tea

Are you struggling to fall asleep at night, and lavender just doesn't do the trick? Try this combination!

Blend these ingredients for 3–4 cups:

- 1 tablespoon of dried chamomile flowers
- 1 tablespoon of dried and crushed lemon balm leaves

With each creation, you learn more about the herbs and how they relate to your body and palate. Whether seeking comfort, health, or simply the pleasure of a delicious cuppa, your tea blends provide a more mindful, enhanced tea experience.

Safety and Precautions

Now, before you unleash your inner herbalist, let's talk safety—ensure your tea blending is not just creative but also smart and safe (*American Herbalists Guild*, 2013):

- **Herb-drug interactions:** Some herbs might not mix well with prescription drugs. For instance, St. John's Wort is a known no-match for blood thinners. Always be sure to check with your healthcare professional before mixing herbs into your daily diet or regimen.
- **Allergy awareness:** Like any new food, herbs can sometimes cause adverse reactions. So, introduce new herbs slowly, monitor your body's response, and listen to any warnings it gives.
- **Pregnancy considerations:** If you're expecting, it's wise to exercise extra caution. Some herbs are not recommended during pregnancy, so when in doubt, it's best to err on the side of caution.

For peace of mind, always keep the lines of communication open with your healthcare practitioner. To guarantee that your tea blending experience is delightful and risk-free, taking a few simple precautions may go a long way. Now that you have these suggestions have fun making your own personal tea blends!

Embracing Herbal Teas in Daily Life

As we reach the end of this chapter, like the last soothing sips of your favorite infusion, we're wrapped up in the cozy glimmer of new wisdom. This section has been an open door to delight in a cup that's both a nod to age-old customs and your health. We've gone through the mysteries of herbal blends, and now, with a clear understanding of each plant's profile, you're ready to craft your own herbal combinations. May your cup brim with joy and your heart with peace as you savor your tea.

Chapter 5

Beyond Teas

Other Ways to Use Herbs

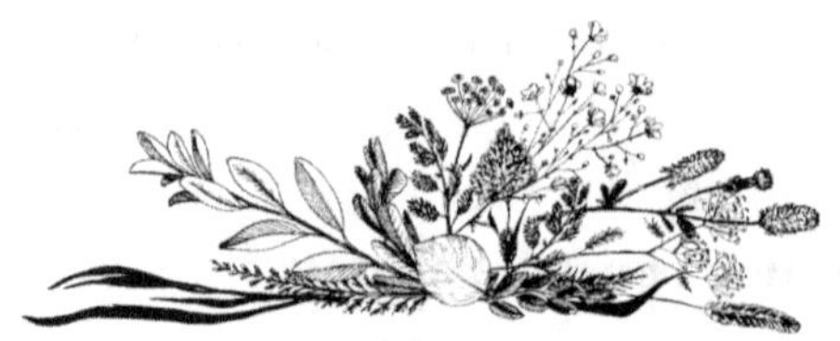

It is my body, my health, my balance, and my responsibility to make the right choices for myself. Right choices include working with competent health-care professionals when necessary, allowing friends and family to help as needed, and, above all, being true to my beliefs, with the wisdom and willingness to change as part of the path of healing.

— Rosemary Gladstar

Think of your favorite tea—maybe it's that peppermint blend that warms you up after a chilly afternoon or the chamomile that's a standby when you need to wind down. Now, imagine stepping out of your comfort zone and into a world where those same herbs can do so much more!

In this chapter, we're not just steeping leaves; we're transforming herbs into a whole cabinet of healing tools. It's like turning your kitchen into a mini lab, but way more fun and without the need for white coats or safety goggles. You'll gently simmer a salve that could soothe your sunburn or the meticulous drip of a tincture tailor-made to ease your friend's relentless allergies. We're about to get hands-on with some of the most incredible, practical DIY herbal magic (yes, magic—because sometimes it feels pretty close to it when that home-made lip balm works wonders). Here's to the excitement of turning what you've grown or bought into your very own line of personal care products. Let's get started, shall we?

Herbal Prospects: Tinctures, Salves, and More

Who knew that your humble herb collection could do so much? Well, the trusty plants that flavor your tea can also be the heroes in various other healthful concoctions. In this part of the chapter, we'll show the practical and somewhat enchanting process of turning your herbal allies into different preparations —each with its unique charm and specific use (Chappell, 2019; Fletcher, 2019).

Tinctures

Imagine capturing the essence of your garden's vitality in just a few drops. That's the essence of a tincture! These herbal powerhouses are created by submerging finely chopped herbs in alcohol or vinegar, releasing their full-bodied benefits into a concentrated extract. After several weeks, once you strain the herbs, you're left with a pure shelf-essence. Their ideal for preserving those delicate plant compounds we've come to cherish, tinctures provide us with wellness in each drop, whether it's to support our digestive health or to calm a restless mind.

Salves

When your skin yearns for relief, turn to salves—the herbal world's soothing embrace. By infusing oils with the healing properties of herbs and setting the mixture with beeswax, you create a spreadable, protective balm. Whether it's for a stubborn scar or a bothersome bug bite, salves are an excellent direct application of nature's care. Plus, getting crafty with your own salves allows you to control the consistency and therapeutic properties. Don't forget to perform a patch test with your homemade salve to make sure your skin is compatible.

Poultices

Poultices are the time-honored tradition of applying raw herbs directly to the skin, a practice that invites the healing energy of nature to address our areas of concern. Whether it's a mash of freshly picked plantain for a bee sting or a warm chamomile paste to soothe those sore muscles after a straining workout, poultices offer us direct relief by combining the raw qualities of herbs with the body's own healing mechanisms. Keep your poultices simple and fresh, and use them to complement your body's natural healing processes.

Infused Oils

The alchemy of transforming herbs into infused oils is a gentle process of coaxing out the lipid-soluble constituents. Whether it's lavender for relaxation or arnica for bruises, these oils become the foundation for many herbal products. Preparing your own means, you can choose the strength and scent, tailoring them to your needs or desires. When creating your infusions, choose a high-quality carrier oil and let the mixture steep in a warm, sunny spot to maximize those herbal benefits.

Herbal Vinegar

Herbal vinegars might be the most versatile performers in your herbal lineup. More than a tangy addition to salads, they're a medium for wellness, rich in minerals, and perfect as a digestive aid or a heart-healthy tonic. Keen to try it at home? Infuse apple cider vinegar with herbs like dandelion or nettle, and you'll have a tonic that's as delicious as it is beneficial. Start with a simple recipe, and experiment with different herbs to find the flavor profiles and health benefits that serve you best.

Hopefully, this section inspired you to explore the various uses of herbs! With each creation, you'll become more adept at transforming your greens into something that fits your lifestyle. So, here's to the craft of herbal preparation—equal parts science, intuition, and a dash of intuitive charm.

Basic DIY Herbal Recipes for Common Ailments

In this section, we'll explore some foundational recipes that transform everyday herbs into influential allies against everyday ailments. From relaxing minor discomforts to freeing you from stress, these DIY recipes are designed to be accessible and effective for any budding herbalist (*Healthline*, 2017; *Rosemary Gladstar's Science & Art of Herbalism*, 2016).

Herbal Tincture for Digestive Health

Are you having some stomach discomfort? This tincture might do the trick. Take 1–2 teaspoons of the tincture before meals to help digestion.

The Green Glow

Ingredients:

- 1 part dried peppermint leaves
- 1 part dried fennel seeds
- 1 part dried ginger root
- vodka or apple cider vinegar for an alcohol-free alternative

Instructions:

1. Combine the herbs in a clean glass jar.
2. Fill the jar with vodka or vinegar until the herbs are completely submerged.
3. Seal the jar and store it in a cool, dark place for 4–6 weeks, shaking it daily.
4. After the steeping period, strain the liquid through a cheesecloth or fine mesh and store it in a clean, dark glass bottle.

Gentle Calendula Salve for Skin Irritations

If you need a natural remedy for minor cuts, scrapes, or dry skin areas, apply this calendula salve for a soothing effect.

Ingredients:

- 1 cup calendula-infused oil, which is created by steeping dried calendula petals in a carrier oil like olive or almond oil for 2–4 weeks
- 1/4 cup beeswax pellets

Instructions:

1. Gently melt the beeswax in a double boiler.

2. Once melted, add the calendula-infused oil and stir until well combined.
3. Remove from heat and pour into small, sterilized jars.
4. Let it cool and set before sealing the jars.

Ginger Poultice for Muscle Aches

You had a tough run or strenuous workout, and you need relief! This ginger poultice does wonders for sore muscles or aches.

Ingredients:

- fresh ginger root
- hot
- a clean cloth or gauze

Instructions:

1. Grate a sufficient amount of fresh ginger root.
2. Soak the grated ginger in hot water for a few minutes.
3. Place the soaked ginger onto the cloth and fold it to make a poultice.
4. Apply the poultice to the affected area for 15–20 minutes.

Chamomile and Lavender Sleep Aid Spray

A restful night's sleep is only a spritz away! Spray this mix onto your pillow and linens before bed to promote relaxation and ensure a good night's sleep.

Ingredients:

- 1 cup distilled water
- 2 tablespoons of dried chamomile flowers

The Green Glow

- 2 tablespoons of dried lavender flowers
- spray bottle

Instructions:

1. Boil the distilled water and pour over the chamomile
   and lavender flowers.
2. Let the mixture steep until it cools down to room
   temperature.
3. Strain the mixture to remove the flowers.
4. Pour the liquid into a spray bottle and apply as
   needed before bedtime.

Thyme and Honey Cough Syrup

Feeling the mid-winter sniffles and occasional cough? All you
need is one tablespoon of this natural cough syrup.

Ingredients:

- 1/4 cup dried thyme leaves
- 1 cup water
- 1 cup honey

Instructions:

1. Boil the water and pour over the thyme leaves,
   allowing it to steep until it cools.
2. Strain the thyme leaves and combine the infused
   water with honey in a saucepan.
3. Heat gently, stirring until the honey and thyme water
   are well combined.
4. Store the mixture in a clean glass bottle.

Safety First: Precautions in Herbal Preparations

As we've already realized, with blending teas, the natural world demands a thoughtful approach. Let's level up that conversation for the more concentrated forms of herbal magic you're working on within this chapter. While some herbs might seem as harmless as a garden party, remember that when concentrated into tinctures, oils, and salves, their potency magnifies (*Better Health Channel*, 2021).

Here are some safety tips to keep in mind for when you start crafting your own recipes:

- **Precision in dosage:** Consider this your measuring mantra: "Start low, go slow." Precision in dosage is critical, especially when a little goes a long way.
- **Spotting sensitive reactions:** Test a patch of skin or start with a tiny dose and wait to see if your body has any new sensations. Your body's feedback is precious; don't ignore the warning signs.
- **Medication mingle-management:** Medications and herbs can have a complicated relationship. Some enhance each other's effects; others might clash. It's best to introduce them cautiously and under the proper guidance, so if you're feeling unsure, it's best to ask your healthcare provider.
- **Quality and source verification:** Sourcing herbs should be done diligently. The origin, purity, and preparation of your herbs can make or break the safety and efficacy of your remedies.

- **Vulnerable populations:** The very young, the elderly, pregnant and nursing individuals, and those with chronic conditions often need gentler, more considered herbal approaches. In these cases, extra care isn't optional; it's essential.
- **Keeping remedies fresh:** Your homegrown remedies aren't eternal. They need the right conditions to preserve their potency and still be safe. Ensure proper storage for longevity.
- **Continuous education:** Herbal knowledge isn't stagnant; it grows and evolves. Stay informed and up-to-date. Good practices today might be outdated tomorrow, so stay on your toes and keep learning!

The world of herbal remedies is enchanting, but it comes with responsibilities. Your role as an herbalist is part alchemist, part scientist—measuring, testing, and respecting the knowledge of nature at your fingertips. Handle your herbs and practice with care, and you will flourish!

Multi-purpose Herbs and Their Preparations

Isn't it astonishing how a few plants from your garden or windowsill can turn into a full-scale wellness toolkit? The simplicity of preparing these natural remedies makes them accessible to everyone, from the novice cook to the seasoned herbalist.

Here's how we can create our own home remedies from some everyday versatile herbs with minimal effort (Fletcher, 2019; *Healthline*, 2017):

- **Turmeric:** Blend turmeric powder, water, and black pepper to create a paste that fights off inflammation.
- **Garlic:** Infuse garlic cloves in oil over low heat to make a versatile remedy with powerful antibacterial benefits.
- **Peppermint:** Make peppermint oil by steeping dried, crushed leaves in oil for its digestive and cooling properties.
- **Echinacea:** Prepare a tincture by soaking the herb in alcohol to enhance your immune defense.
- **Ginger:** Simmer slices of ginger root in water to make a soothing tea that can aid digestion and reduce nausea.
- **Cinnamon:** Stir cinnamon sticks in warm water or add powdered cinnamon to dishes for its blood sugar-regulating and antimicrobial effects.
- **Thyme:** Create a thyme infusion by steeping the leaves in hot water, which can be used as a throat gargle for its antiseptic properties.
- **Basil:** Steep fresh basil leaves in hot water to create a tea that may alleviate stress and stomach discomfort.
- **Sage:** Boil sage leaves and let them steep to make a strong infusion that can be used as a mouthwash for its antibacterial properties.
- **Lemon balm:** Combine fresh lemon balm leaves with vodka to create a tincture that could help reduce anxiety and promote sleep.

With these effortless preparations, you can get the significant benefits of these plants right in the comfort of your home. Have fun exploring with them!

Healing Is in Your Hands

This chapter emphasizes the enchanting abilities of herbs in advancing our health and wellness. We now know that herbalism is not limited to teas but can be applied to various practices, such as creating tinctures and salves.

Cultivating self-reliance and celebrating each successful remedy as a personal triumph in exploring natural health is essential. The satisfaction of each small victory fuels your passion for learning and growing as an herbalist. By mixing nature's ingredients, we blend tradition with innovation, science with art, and plants with purpose. You can step forward with confidence, knowing that your healing hands can transform the way you care for yourself and your loved ones. The herbs are ready, the knowledge is set, and the natural, healthy life you desire is yours.

Chapter 6

Integrating Herbalism Into Daily Life

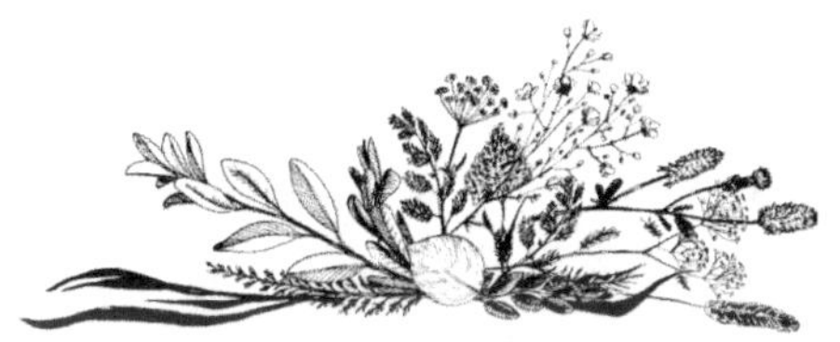

Herbs are the friend of the physician and the pride of cooks.

— Charlemagne

Within the gentle flow of our daily activities, there's an understated yet impactful chance to merge the healing qualities of herbs into our familiar patterns. Herbal practices don't have to be isolated to times of illness or deliberate health pursuits; they can be as routine and constant as the dawn cycle to dusk. This chapter invites you to understand how the ancient knowledge of herbs can seamlessly interact with your day-to-day life, from the aromatic steam of your morning brew to the calming lotion you apply before sleep. Welcome the transition to a lifestyle where your selection of spices also serves as a collection of remedies, and cooking becomes an act of nurturing well-being. Here, we engage in a natural partnership with the environment, welcoming its benefits into our homes, lives, and ordinary experiences. Welcome to the natural inclusion of herbal practices in your life—a journey toward wellness and an enriched bond with the pace of the natural world (Hoshaw, 2021).

Daily Routines With an Herbal Twist

Herbs can be a simple way of improving health and vitality when included in daily routines. The key is to integrate herbal benefits naturally into your day-to-day activities. Below are suggestions for bringing the vitality of herbs into your routine (NT Contributor, 2003; Sullivan, 2020):

- **Morning awakening:** Begin your day by gently stimulating your body and mind with herbal alternatives. Trade your coffee for a revitalizing herbal tea like ginseng or peppermint; this means no more morning jitters from too much caffeine! Ginseng offers a natural boost to your central nervous system, promoting mental focus and energy without the crash associated with caffeine. Peppermint tea greets you with a refreshing zing, stimulates digestion, and helps clear morning fog.
- **Culinary creations:** Make your meals an opportunity to introduce herbs that not only enrich flavor but also offer health benefits. Mix fresh cilantro into your guacamole for a detoxifying twist, or blend sage into your butter for an aromatic spread that boosts both memory and taste.
- **Mindful self-care:** Rejuvenate your skincare practice with herbal products. Expand beyond aloe vera to include rose petals for moisture, healing calendula, and toning witch hazel. Design skincare

treatments suited to your needs, like a green tea mist for antioxidant protection or a neem leaf soak for its purifying qualities, or you can start with something simple like adding a few drops of lavender oil to your moisturizer.

- **Clean and green:** Transform your cleaning routine by making your herbal solutions. Try rosemary-infused vinegar for a cleanser that clears the mind with its aroma. Combine one part rosemary-infused vinegar with two parts water for an effective and all-natural surface cleaner. Discover the antifungal benefits of thyme by using it in a lemon-thyme mixture to clean windows and brighten your living space with its uplifting scent.
- **Evening wind-down:** As the evening approaches, encourage relaxation with herbs known for their calming effects. Introduce a pre-sleep ritual with teas like skullcap and lemon balm to ease into restfulness. For some aromatic comfort, add hop flowers to a small pillow or sleep sachet to promote a peaceful night's sleep.

When we include these herbal routines in our lives, we create an environment that benefits our health and happiness. How will you choose to work herbs into your day-to-day routine?

Herbs for Everyday

How else can we invite more of nature into our day? Here, we discover some unique, underrated herbs that can improve sleep quality, support digestive health, and help us manage stress better (*American Herbal Pharmacopoeia*, 2023; Sullivan, 2020).

For Peaceful Slumbers

When the night comes, and sleep doesn't come easily, nature's own selection of herbs can be a gentle solution. Here are two botanicals other than lavender and chamomile that can help you achieve a peaceful night's sleep, enhancing your bedtime routine with their calming properties:

- **Passionflower (*Passiflora incarnata*):** This plant is not only visually striking but also holds compounds that could assist in combating insomnia. Prepare tea from the dried leaves and flowers for a calming pre-sleep drink. Enjoy it about an hour before bed, letting its gentle floral essence set the stage for relaxation.
- **Hops (*Humulus lupulus*):** Beyond their use in the beer industry, hops have qualities that can contribute to a good night's sleep. Although their bitter taste may not be suitable for tea, placing a small pouch of dried hops near your pillow can be soothing, as their fragrance is thought to promote sleep.

For Digestive Harmony

We can't deny that a well-functioning digestive system is fundamental to our overall well-being, and the botanical world offers critical ingredients for its care. Below are more herbs that can gently restore digestive balance, offering natural and palatable solutions.

- **Lemon balm (*Melissa officinalis*):** This herb, with its inviting citrus fragrance, can help soothe digestive discomfort. For a cold infusion, steep the leaves in cool water for a few hours and drink throughout the day. It is incredibly refreshing when your digestion needs a gentle boost.

- **Dandelion root (*Taraxacum officinale*):** Often dismissed as a simple lawn weed, dandelion root is excellent for digestion. A tea made from roasted dandelion root serves as a mild liver tonic, aiding in digestion and providing a rich, coffee-like taste without caffeine.

Add a teaspoon of honey if you like your beverages on the sweeter side.

For Stress Relief

Ah, yes. Stress is an inevitable part of modern life, but nature provides a way to mitigate its effects. We highlight some uncommon herbs that offer a calming influence on our minds and strengthen the body's resilience:

- **Holy basil (*Ocimum sanctum*):** Known in Ayurvedic practice as Tulsi, this herb is celebrated for its adaptogenic qualities, which help the body to better adapt to stress. Keep a small jar of holy basil on your desk; simply open it and take a deep breath. It can be a quick stress reliever during a hectic day! A warm cup of holy basil tea can be deeply soothing, as its aromatic profile helps to rebalance stress levels.
- **Ashwagandha (*Withania somnifera*):** The roots of ashwagandha, with their distinctive earthy taste, are ideal in a warm, milky mixture before bed or as a morning supplement in its powder form. It is traditionally revered for strengthening the nervous system and stress resilience.

The skill of using herbs effectively is to combine them thoughtfully into your daily habits. Let this guide encourage you to broaden your knowledge and use herbal remedies for a well-balanced approach to natural health.

Mindfulness in Herbal Practice: Cultivating Intuition

In the nurturing space of herbalism, mindfulness is akin to the light that fosters our bond with plant partners, enhancing both their effectiveness and our understanding of them. Developing intuition in this field is about nurturing a unique relationship with herbs that expands beyond their recognized applications. It involves paying attention to the little things—noticing how your body reacts to different herbs and the insights that emerge in moments of quiet and focus. Introducing specific herbal recipes designed to enhance intuition can amplify this mindfulness practice. For instance, preparing a blend of dried blue lotus flower, lavender, and chamomile for tea or a bath can be a deeply meditative process, allowing for a serene state in which one's intuition may flourish (Cassie, 2020; *Matthew Wood Institute of Herbalism*, 2023; Pande, 2021).

Herbal Meditation Practices

Within the quiet of meditation, herbs such as calming blue lotus, lavender, and chamomile become more than supplements; they connect us to heightened awareness. The methodical preparation of these herbs into tea becomes a ritual, fostering a space where mindfulness and intuition intersect. As one ingests the tea or immerses oneself in a bath infused with these ingredients, there is an opening for the calmness required for intuitive work (Cassie, 2020). This practice of intuitive herbalism is about being entirely present with the effect the herb has on your internal experience.

Journaling Your Herbal Experiences

Accompany your sensory explorations with a journal, turning herbal practices into a journey of self-discovery. When journaling, one might reflect on the calming influence of an intuition tea or the protective aura of a mugwort and lavender smoke blend. These experiences, along with the immediate physical reactions and deeper emotional responses, build a comprehensive guide to your herbal intuition journey. Don't know where to start with journaling? Begin by listing the herbs you've used each day and any changes in mood or energy you felt.

Guided Meditation Scripts

To further enhance our intuitive connection with herbs, guided meditation scripts can focus on the qualities of specific plants, like the protective nature of cedarwood or the clarity provided by rosemary and peppermint, both of which have been associated with the third eye chakra and intuitive work (Cassie, 2020; Weed, 2023). Through these meditations, we can explore the plants' symbolic and literal influences on their mindfulness practice.

Interactive Exercises to Engage the Senses

Interactive exercises, such as creating personalized sprays for intuition with essential oils of rosemary, peppermint, and cedarwood, allow for a multi-sensory engagement that can enhance your intuitive abilities, so be sure to spritz some whenever you need a boost of clarity. These sprays can clear the mind and inspire before undertaking intuitive practices (Cassie, 2020). Such hands-on activities not only create a product for further mindfulness but also deepen the intuitive dialogue between practitioner and herb (Hoshaw, 2021).

Aligning With Natural Rhythms

Harmonizing with natural rhythms is enriched by the use of herbs that correspond to these cycles. For instance, the new moon's sense of beginning can be enhanced by the energizing essence of rosemary, while the full moon's culmination might resonate better with the tranquility of chamomile. Using specific herbs in sync with lunar and seasonal changes encourages a reconnection with ancient wisdom and the cycles of the natural world, thereby encouraging an environment where your intuition can grow (Cassie, 2020; Pande, 2021).

Each sip of intuition tea, each breath in a meditative space scented by an intuition smoke blend, and each spritz of an intuitive spray becomes an opportunity to deepen our mindful connection with our inner self and the natural world.

Your Herbal Wellness Plan

You might be feeling unsure of where to start, so here's a roadmap. Begin by selecting the foundational herbs that support your daily wellness. Opt for peppermint to refresh your mornings and sharpen your focus, and consider nettles to enrich your body with vital nutrients. Then, add adaptogens to your routine to cultivate balance and strength. Schisandra berry, in particular, offers dual benefits, boosting your stress resilience and supporting liver function. Gotu kola is excellent when you need cognitive support, especially during the mental exertion needed to complete that project before the deadline or to study for an upcoming exam!

As the day winds down, embrace rituals that promote restoration. Enjoy oat straw tea, a mild nerve tonic, to transition into calmness. On nights when sleep seems just out of reach, a small dose of *Rhodiola rosea* tincture can aid in establishing healthy sleep cycles, ensuring you wake up refreshed and ready for the day ahead.

Think of your wellness approach as a dynamic guide that grows and adjusts with you. Consistently evaluate and adjust your herbal choices to align with your needs (*David Winston's Center for Herbal Studies*, 2023). Be sure to keep a record of how each herb affects you, fine-tuning your daily practices to create a wellness routine that is personal to you.

Living in Harmony With Herbs

As we reach the end of this chapter, I hope that you feel inspired to integrate the herbal knowledge you've gained into your lifestyle with more peace of mind. Consider the subtle strengths of lesser-known herbs, such as the stress-relieving lemon balm or the resilient ashwagandha, which can support you through life's changes, such as the curveballs and unexpected events we can't possibly plan for.

Allow these insights to help you thrive on a personal journey of becoming one with nature. Welcome the embrace of the herbal world, and let your life be enhanced by the sheer delight of connecting with your botanicals.

Chapter 7

The Broader World of Herbalism
Future and Community

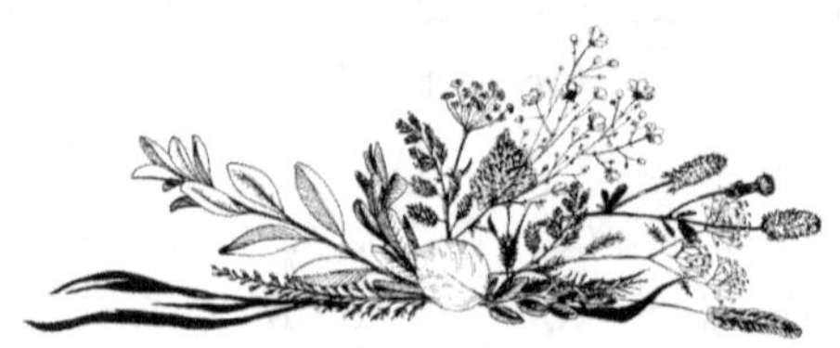

Herbs are the gentle healers of the world.

— Barbara Griggs

Herbs have long been recognized as "gentle healers of the world," and this chapter zeroes in on the expanding influence of herbalism from intimate community roots to its place in the global setting. We glimpse how herbal practices encourage community well-being, evolve through education, and prosper through sustainable and technological innovation.

The chapter discusses the growing recognition of herbal medicine in society and the pivotal role of education in shaping knowledgeable practitioners. It underscores the importance of sustainable and ethical practices in the industry and highlights the interconnectedness of herbalists worldwide in preserving and evolving the craft.

Technological advancements are acknowledged for propelling herbalism into the future alongside the essential community spirit that bolsters the field through symposiums, mentorship, and advocacy.

In essence, this chapter imagines a future in which herbalism combines established practices with cutting-edge research to preserve its modern relevance and therapeutic effectiveness. Now, let's find your fellow herbalists!

Strengthening Connections Through Community

At the heart of every community is the intrinsic power of connection and restoration found in herbalism. This section looks into how the tradition of herbal use surpasses mere health benefits, becoming a crucial aspect of cultural identity within community gardens. We explore how herbalism is intertwined with individual health and the collective vitality of communities worldwide (Vasilis, 2023). Remember when you stumbled on your local herbal workshop and walked away with a new favorite remedy for easing your nerves? It's these small discoveries that enhance our daily wellness practices!

So, how can we then strengthen our connections through community?

Local beginnings and community building:

- Beginnings are often marked by casual gatherings or workshops where herbal secrets and remedies are shared, validating long-standing traditions and knowledge. This might just be where you find the

recipe for your new favorite tincture! Practical wisdom passed from neighbor to neighbor.
- These small, intimate settings provide the foundation for larger endeavors, nurturing a space where personal stories and expertise flourish and grow.

The global expansion of herbalism through digital platforms:

- Platforms like Instagram and Facebook have become vibrant corners on the internet for herbalism enthusiasts to exchange guidance, narratives, and safeguards.
- Online communities are vital in enhancing the dialogue of understanding and in establishing strong, supportive networks that span across the globe.
- E-commerce has empowered local herbal practitioners to market their handcrafted products globally, providing them with the economic sustainability of their crafts.

Professional networks and global integration:

- Organizations such as the National Association for Holistic Aromatherapy (NAHA) and American Herbalists Guild (AHG) create opportunities for professional collaboration, keeping their members informed of industry trends and promoting events that blend traditional and modern practices where plant lovers unite and discuss the latest leafy trends!
- These organizations show us the intersection of diverse practices can empower a meaningful global herbal community.

The Evolution and Recognition of Herbal Medicine

Looking back through history, the ancient wisdom surrounding herbs remains influential. There is an increased collective respect and recognition for the role of herbal medicine in managing everyday health. The emerging trend toward more holistic and accessible health practices, mainly the Community Supported Herbal Medicine Movement, represents a societal acceptance of natural remedies as integral to daily wellness (*Stafford Madeer, 2023*).

Educational Pathways in Herbalism

We know that education is essential for developing our expertise, and the same goes for growing our confidence in herbalism. Just as you're now learning what herbalism is, you're expanding your understanding, ensuring the safe and efficient use of herbs; there are renowned organizations like Mountain Rose Herbs that offer comprehensive courses that prepare us to practice herbalism more proficiently. Additionally, ambitions like the Herbalista mobile clinics help share herbal knowledge, enhancing accessibility and community health.

There is a broader range of educational opportunities available for those fascinated by herbalism and who want to uncover more than the foundations:

- **Accredited institutions,** such as the Maryland University of Integrative Health, offer formal programs that blend scientific and traditional knowledge, developing your proficiency in botany, phytochemistry, and clinical application.
- **Professional bodies** like the American Herbalists Guild also advance our professional excellence by

offering certifications that necessitate ongoing education, adherence to the latest research, and other sustainable practices.

Sustainability and Ethical Considerations

Sustainable practices are at the core of responsible herbalism. Gaia Herbs demonstrates this commitment through its dedication to environmental stewardship and ensuring its operations contribute positively to our planet and, so, our personal health. This principle underpins the broader societal role of herbalism, reinforcing the idea that each botanical product should be created with respect for the Mother Nature that provides it (*Gaia Herbs*, 2021).

Connecting With Professional Herbalists and Resources

Connecting with experienced herbalists is crucial for deepening one's understanding of plant-based healing. The American Herbalists Guild, for instance, offers a directory to locate credible herbalists and endorses reliable online retailers, thus guaranteeing that the quality of herbs procured is a matter of informed choice (Hoshaw, 2021).

Lifelong Learning: Advanced Studies and Specialization

There is so much more to this art! The field of herbalism encourages endless learning and possibilities for specialization. Initial education might begin with basic courses, like an Herb 101 class, from local schools or online platforms such as The Herbal Medicine Academy that allow for flexible learning. However, your educational journey could continually advance into more specialized fields like clinical herbalism or ethnobotany, encompassing extensive coursework, clinical experience, and research masterclasses.

Herbalism in the Public Sphere

The synergy of herbalism with conservation initiatives is signified by entities like United Plant Savers, whose mission exceeds preserving native medicinal plants to ingraining the understanding and use of these plants within our societal perspectives. They advocate for and implement sustainable harvesting methods that are crucial to maintaining the biodiversity that serves as the foundation of our herbalism practices (*United Plant Savers*, 2022).

Their advocacy reaches into policy and education, emphasizing the importance of plant-based remedies to legislators and arguing for the right to practice herbalism without excessive restrictions. This advocacy takes on heightened significance in a world where striking a balance between human needs and the integrity of nature is increasingly fragile.

Organizations like United Plant Savers are much needed in local education, delivering workshops and producing materials stimulating our eco-conscious engagement with plant life. We need to take better care of our planet and the life that inhabits it, and this includes plants!

Practical Engagement With Herbalism

How do we apply all of this knowledge to building or sustaining a thriving community practically? Active involvement and connectivity with the herbalism community can be achieved through various hands-on experiences:

- **Participate in workshops and plant identification walks:** Does your neighborhood or city have regular plant days? Consider joining local events that provide invaluable knowledge from experienced herbalists. It can be an excellent venue for experiential learning, community networking, and a way to make eco-minded friends!
- **Attend herbalism conferences:** These gatherings usually offer a wealth of current research and methodologies, keeping practitioners, such as ourselves, up-to-date on advancements within the herbalism discipline.
- **Engage with community gardens:** Ready to get your hands dirty? Direct experience growing and gathering herbs guided by educational programs on herb recognition and crafting herbal preparations is priceless.

Here is how you can go the extra mile to incorporate herbs into your daily routine besides by practicing the art:

- **Harness educational materials:** A vast collection of books and digital content that caters to diverse interests within herbalism, assisting in the awareness and implementation of its principles.
- **Connect with online herbalism groups:** Digital forums and social media groups centered on herbalism provide a wealthy source of guidance, shared experiences, and communal support. Don't be afraid to ask them how they made that enchanting herbal-infused tea.
- **Take part in interactive herb databases:** These tools are invaluable for researching various

herbs and their applications and are beneficial for educational and practical exercises. Perfect for settling those "What's this plant?" debates.

By actively participating in these initiatives and harnessing the available tools, we can meaningfully weave herbalism into our lifestyle, improving our personal health, supporting sustainable practices, and developing a stronger connection to the natural world. Who knew going green could be so much fun?

Planting Seeds for the Future

What about future generations? Educational programs oriented toward younger people are essential to maintain the cultural relevance of our herbal practices.

These initiatives might include:

- **Herbal education in schools:** Integrating herbal studies into existing curricula to give students a foundation in botanical knowledge.
- **Interactive youth programs:** Implementing programs in botanical gardens and nature reserves that engage children and teens with the natural world.

The Herb Society of America is among the organizations that provide scholarships and materials to encourage youth interest in herbalism and offer summer programs, internships, and workshops to nurture an appreciation for plant traditions and the environment.

Below are other ways we can cultivate a brighter future for herbalism:

Sustainable Practices for Herbal Stewardship

- **Ethical cultivation:** Embracing practices that ensure the long-term viability of herbal plants, particularly endangered ones. Be sure to read which herbs are on the list (United Plant Savers, 2022). Here are a few on the "at-risk" and "to-watch" lists: American Ginseng (*Panax quinquefolius*), Black Cohosh (*Actaea racemosa*), Echinacea (*Echinacea spp.*), Eyebright (*Euphrasia spp.*), Goldenseal (*Hydrastis canadensis*), Slippery Elm (*Ulmus rubra*).
- **Industry responsibility:** Prioritizing habitat conservation, organic farming, and fair trade to meet increasing herbal product demands responsibly (*American Herbal Products Association*, 2022).
- **Eco-friendly packaging:** Using renewable resources in product packaging and distribution to reduce environmental impact. Hello, paper plates, bamboo cups, and glass jars!

Collaborative Efforts

- **Interdisciplinary strategies:** Working with conservationists and agricultural experts to create a sustainable balance between business interests and ecological health.
- **Conservation initiatives:** Establishing herb sanctuaries, seed banks, and breeding programs to secure the survival of at-risk plant species.

As an herbalist enthusiast, you can support ecological health by partnering with local conservationists and gardeners to promote sustainable herb cultivation and help establish community seed libraries or gardens that preserve "at-risk" plants.

Advancing Herbalism With Technology

- **Digital tools:** Try apps like PictureThis or iNaturalist for plant identification, and look for lab analysis features within them to judge herbal quality.
- **Scientific research:** Keep updated with the latest studies on herbal efficacy by checking databases such as PubMed or following the Journal of Herbal Medicine.
- **Supply chain integrity:** Blockchain for supply chain ensures that each step from plant harvesting to your shelf is recorded and can be traced back for authenticity; companies like Provenance and VeChain are examples of platforms offering this technology.

Community and Synergy as Central Pillars

The herbalism community thrives on its unity and shared knowledge!

- **Symposiums and celebrations:** Partake in events like the International Herb Symposium or local herb festivals that celebrate plant medicine and bring enthusiasts together.
- **Mentorship programs:** Look for apprenticeships or mentorship opportunities with established herbalists through organizations like the American Herbalists Guild or regional herbalism schools.
- **Public health integration:** Get involved by advocating for the inclusion of herbal options at local

health clinics or wellness centers and participating in public forums to discuss the benefits of integrating herbal medicine.

The future of herbalism hinges on both preserving ancient wisdom through education and embracing sustainable and technological advances, ensuring this practice remains relevant and beneficial for generations to come.

Cultivating an Herbal Legacy

As we come to the end of our exploration through herbalism, it becomes evident that the healing potential of plants has not withered over time. The number of herbalists, enthusiasts, and supporters is increasing as more people come to understand the immense value of herbal knowledge.

Herbalism has an extensive history as a therapeutic art, and its continued success depends on the care and attention given to this community, respect for tradition, and openness to new ideas. You can help make the world a better place by doing what you can at home, in your community, and through advocacy for transformation.

Together, we have the opportunity and responsibility to manage this garden of knowledge and create a lasting legacy that will serve as a source of energy and motivation for our future generations.

Conclusion
Your Herbal Journey Ahead

In a way, magic is the act of making a wish come about.
Like praying, like plotting, like herbs, like exerting your
will on the world, making something happen.

— Philippa Gregory

In the quiet moments following the end of *An Introduction to Herbalism*, it becomes clear that the final sentence is not a period but a comma, signaling a brief pause before leading to an open door of further exploration. This guide, with its comprehensive chapters, has laid out the fundamentals of herbalism, threading together time-honored herbal wisdom with the growing need for holistic health practices in our modern world.

From unraveling the complexities of plant chemistry to offering sage advice on how you can cultivate your own garden and effectively create your own herb remedies, this guide has inspired the variety of ways nature can become part of our daily lives and help restore a sense of balance that is so easily lost during the rush of "getting things done."

Now, with this foundational knowledge, the invitation goes beyond this last page. You are not just a reader anymore but a practitioner encouraged to step into the living practice of herbalism. This book serves as your beginning to a green way of living, nudging you to craft your own course through the expanding fields of herbal remedies. How will your herbal story unfold? Will you seek out a like-minded community in your midst or advocate for a more natural way of living online?

This ongoing process of discovery and sharing has the potential to spark a collective awakening and encourage more and more individuals to reconnect with the natural world, and the wellness it offers is endless!

As you create your own innovations, be it a unique tea blend, a soothing balm, or a tincture, by sharing your insights, you contribute to a collective understanding, maintaining a community that values health, sustainability, and respect for the living world. The story of herbalism is ever-unfolding, and you are now a part of it.

Standing at this entryway, consider the paths before you. Take a moment to reflect on your journey through these pages. How has your perspective shifted? What practices resonate most with you? How will you do more of that? Your personal reflections will guide your steps as you grow into your role as an herbalist.

To further your learning and engagement with herbalism and to join a community where every voice matters, consider this your exclusive invitation to our vibrant Facebook group,

"Herbs, Hearts, and Healing." This group is a gathering space for those who share a passion for nature's wisdom and a commitment to wellness. Our rapidly growing community is a cornerstone of our brand, offering you the unique opportunity to connect with fellow herbal enthusiasts, exchange your ideas, and receive a boost of motivation on your journey. By joining, you become part of an inspiring community dedicated to exploring the endless opportunities that herbal remedies bring. A world of support and shared knowledge is just a click away! Witness your herbal practice thrive among friends.

Thank you for embracing The Green Glow as your ally on this enlightening expedition into herbalism. May you continue to nurture this bond with the healing herbs of the Earth and find your healthiest, most vibrant self. As our guide concludes, consider leaving a review to share how this journey has impacted you. What lessons will you carry with you as you continue your practice? Your feedback is valuable as it not only helps us improve and refine but also allows others to find their own path in the natural healing embrace of herbalism.

A final thought: Continuously seek out new information, be open to change, and adapt as science and traditions evolve. May your path be magical and evergreen!

How to Grow Your Own Medicine

The Ultimate Beginner's Guide to Holistic Healing with Natural Remedies and Medicinal Herbs

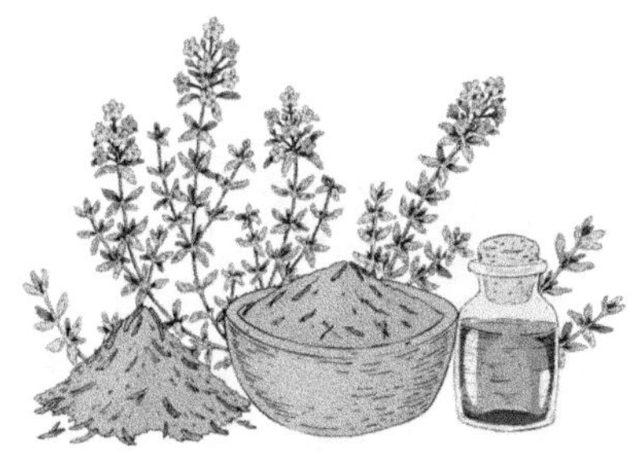

Introduction

"I know of nothing else in medicine that can come close to what a plant-based diet can do. In theory, if everyone were to adopt this, I really believe we can cut health care costs by seventy to eighty percent. That's amazing. And it all comes from understanding nutrition, applying nutrition, and just watching the results."

— *T. Colin Campbell*

Plants have provided food and medicine to mankind for thousands of years. Early humans discovered that several common plants had potent medicinal qualities through close observation and generational knowledge transfer. This is how a great deal of the powerful medications used in contemporary medicine were initially discovered in nature. By learning about herbs, you can support your well-being through easily accessible natural remedies, as those before us did, while maintaining valuable wisdom and resources for all.

Since the beginning of settled human communities, people have relied on nature's plentiful plants to treat various health issues. Across all regions and eras, herbal medicines from accessible native species served as the main form of medical care available. Many drugs commonly used now actually originated as the isolated active components of those very same healing herbs known for centuries: Aspirin from willow, morphine from poppies, and quinine from cinchona bark. Even with sophisticated modern options, plants remain hugely significant to global healthcare, with recent statistics showing over 25% of prescribed pharmaceuticals contain plant-derived chemical constituents as their key ingredients (Fields, 2016). This underscores how humanity's long relationship with nurturing knowledge from the land remains deeply intertwined with supporting worldwide wellness today.

Over the last century, as modern medicine has advanced, many people have lost touch with the healing plants that sustained communities for millennia. Today, most turn primarily to physicians when ill instead of using readily available natural remedies. However, cultivating knowledge of beneficial native species offers advantages such as greater self-sufficiency, sustainability, and potentially lower healthcare costs. This book aims to rediscover the deep history and wisdom of herbalism by practically teaching the cultivation of medicinal plants you can grow yourself. By learning herbal traditions passed down through generations, you can tap into readily accessible natural solutions, support overall wellness, and potentially complement treatment from physicians. Reconnecting with flora's therapeutic benefits offers empowerment to nurture well-being through a more connected relationship with the land, as people have throughout history.

This book provides a complete course to cultivate valuable medicinal plant skills, taking you from beginner gardener to knowledgeable herbal practitioner. Clear instructions teach you to select species suited to your climate, propagate from seeds, care for growth, and properly harvest. Learn identification methods to ensure the use of the right plants, as well as save seeds for future use. Discover ideal growing conditions customized for each variety. Most importantly, detailed preparation, ratio, and testing methods are covered to create safe remedies like teas, extracts, ointments, and elixirs from your homegrown materials. Following the step-by-step process empowers self-care through sustainable, natural resources accessible right in your backyard or community. These traditions hold wisdom to support wellness when shared with interested people seeking to improve access to personalized holistic healthcare.

This guide encourages cultivating medicinal plants not only for their practical health benefits but also as a meditative practice. Spending time tending a garden invites slowing your pace, developing stillness, promoting concentration skills, and fostering an appreciation for environmental rhythms. Just as different species flourish or rest across seasons, tending them alongside such natural changes nurtures increased patience. Rather than rushing through tasks, conscious gardening immerses you mindfully in elemental interactions. The earth's renewal mirrors life's passages while working alongside growth cycles, which reflects humanity's small role within vast interconnected webs. This perspective cultivates gratitude, reminding us that sustenance and well-being arise from respectful, attentive participation in the greater whole.

Introduction

Herbalism as mindfulness offers preventative self-care through observant participation in nature's wisdom.

Digging your hands into the earth can do as much good for your mind as your plants. Just digging in the dirt and feeling that cool soil helps you let out a lot of stress and worry. And nothing lifts the spirits like seeing new green growth pop up. As you care for your patch over the seasons, you really get to know each plant—like how hydrangeas look when they are thirsty or how it may be when viburnums are plump and ready. There's a feeling of pride that comes with that deep understanding like you're passing on useful tips to others. Really, tending a little garden connects you to something bigger than yourself. It feels good to be part of the ongoing human story of learning from and caring for the green things that give us life.

Most significantly, maintaining a medicinal garden connects you to a long history of people who cultivated knowledge of healing plants. From early indigenous communities to herbalists throughout history, many contributed valuable lessons that extended accessible natural remedies through eras. Whether discovering properties, cultivating uses, documenting research, or distributing plant-derived drugs, each built upon previous generations' insights into nature's pharmacy. By learning traditional identification, growing practices, and herbal preparations, you become part of safeguarding that legacy and ensuring these benefits continue to be accessible. Brewing your first cup of therapeutic tea reminds you how present-day wellness sits upon foundations laid long ago. Participating in this unbroken chain linking all who treasured and advanced botanical wisdom across time instills an appreciation for deep roots from which future understandings may also grow.

Now, let's begin our journey into the wondrous world of plants as guides, teachers, food, and friends. Turn to Chapter One, and we'll take the first step by assessing our health priorities and selecting powerful medicinal plants to share our gardens with. Soon, you may come to see your new green friends as the wisest doctors of all. The transformed landscape holds life-affirming lessons we have only to listen for. Let the healing begin!

Chapter 1

Introduction to Herbal Medicine

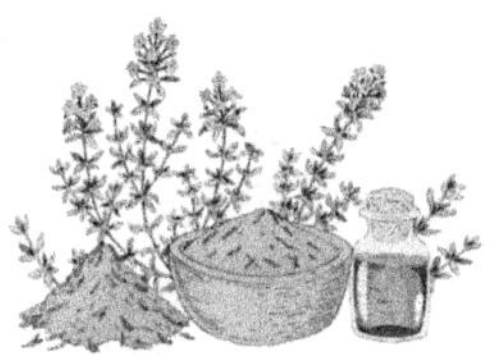

For millennia, people have depended on medicinal plants as a primary source of healthcare. Nearly every civilization cultivated a deep understanding of which native species soothed specific ailments or improved overall well-being. As populations migrated and exchanged goods, familiarity with remedies native to other lands also spread far and wide. Through countless observations, folk wisdom systematically identified which herbs and preparations routinely alleviated sickness and suffering when illnesses inevitably struck individuals and communities. Across changing eras and distant places, collective traditional insights continually reinforced how certain easily accessible botanicals offered reliable relief. Both structured medical systems and grassroots experimentation by healers everywhere steadily expanded knowledge of nature's pharmacy.

Herbalism provides a holistic approach to healthcare, incorporating many natural options. Various plant-based remedies like tinctures, teas, and dried herbs are used alongside dietary and habit changes. Whole herbs contain complex mixtures of organic substances that can interact for healing but also prevent unwanted side effects. In contrast, pharmaceuticals contain only isolated single chemicals and lack the buffers found in full plant preparations. By using complete botanical extracts, herbalism encourages multiple components to work together for benefit. This balance capitalizes on the synergistic interactions inherent in intact materials directly from nature. This systematic yet moderated framework aims to restore wellness gently and sustainably through treatments respectful of our bodies as interconnected with the greater natural world around us.

As modern research increasingly confirms long-held understanding of herbal healthcare, many individuals now seek natural options as complements or alternatives to standard pharmaceutical interventions. No plant is a cure-all, yet becoming familiar with herbal properties empowers you to make choices aligned with personal values and wellness goals. Rather than relying solely on prescriptions or procedures, rediscovering easily accessible botanical remedies as low-risk adjunct supports provides greater self-determination. When combined judiciously with other treatments under guidance, an open but discerning approach allows for both honoring science and tradition. Reconnecting with healing gifts from nature that have supported humanity since time immemorial invites tapping sustainably into what has nourished community health for generations by participating actively in one's care through a cultivated partnership with the living earth around us.

The Ancient Roots

People have used medicinal plants for healthcare since long before any written records existed, with findings showing this practice dates back over 60,000 years (Yuan et al., 2016). All early societies depended greatly on native flora, like certain trees, herbs, flowers, and mushrooms, to treat their sick. Over immense time, various cultures independently developed structured frameworks for applying botanical remedies, laying the groundwork for the medical systems we still acknowledge today. Complex traditional herbal wisdom emerged separately around the globe, illustrating how attentive co-existence with one's surroundings cultivated a deep universal understanding of organic compounds that fortified survival.

Historical Overview

Ancient civilizations around the globe developed herbal pharmacopeias unique to their local flora, climate, and prevalent illnesses. The first herbal compendium dates from over 5000 years ago in Sumer (Pan et al., 2014), followed by Egyptian scrolls and Chinese manuscripts detailing hundreds of medicinal plants. Compilations from India, Greece, Rome, the Middle East, and Europe demonstrate how herbal healing knowledge circulated along early trade routes. As people migrated, they carried plant seeds and remedies to new lands. Through an accumulation of observations and experiences over millennia, generations of indigenous healers and folk practitioners contributed to an expansive catalog of herbal medicine that continues to inform medicine today.

Traditional Healing Systems

Some long-established medical frameworks have especially helped shape modern herbalism. Systems like Ayurveda,

Traditional Chinese Medicine (TCM), and indigenous medicine view health comprehensively, seeing emotional, mental, spiritual, and social well-being as fundamentally linked to physical health. These major medical traditions take a whole-body perspective by combining herbal remedies with minerals aimed at balancing one's inner vital energy and supporting self-healing capacity.

Ayurveda

Emerging at least 3000 years ago in India, Ayurveda aims to harmonize forces of nature and energy within the body through diet, herbs, massage, yoga, and meditation. Diagnosis identifies an individual's predominant doshas (constitutions), and treatment restores balance among *Vata* (air or wind), *Pitta* (fire), and *Kapha* (earth and water) influences. Key herbs like turmeric, ginger, cinnamon, and gotu kola address common complaints.

Traditional Chinese Medicine

An ancient medical system formalized in China by 1000 BCE sees health as a balance between opposing but interdependent energies termed "yin" and "yang." According to this view, *qi* (vital energy) circulates along pathways called "meridians" linked to internal organs. Specific herbs such as ginseng, astragalus, and licorice address imbalances like shortages or disruptions of flow. TCM employs stimulation methods such as acupuncture and massage aimed at restoring homeostasis in the body. By evaluating factors including emotions, environment, and physiology as dynamically linked, TCM's principles highlight an integrated perspective that healthcare arises from respecting life's subtle interconnected rhythms—both within and beyond human form—which herbal and manual stimulation techniques aim to cultivate for overall well-being.

Indigenous Healing Practices

From Australian Aboriginal bush medicine to Native American sweat lodges to Siberian shamans, diverse Indigenous cultures share herbal wisdom and holistic spiritual rituals passed down orally for generations. These rich traditions integrate botanical treatments with ceremony, community support, and reverence for nature's healing power. Herbs offer multidimensional benefits—dandelion for vitality, mullein for cough—while chanting, plant baths, and vision quests connect people with divine curative energy to augment plant medicines.

This time-tested integrative framework underlies contemporary naturopathic approaches to harnessing nature's healing gifts. As herbalism experiences renewed interest worldwide, modern medicine has just begun to tap into the therapeutic potential of plants when used synergistically and holistically.

Herbal Medicine in Contemporary Health

Following a time when medical practices in Western nations centered increasingly on technology and pharmaceuticals, interest in herbalism is currently growing as many individuals pursue more comprehensive, natural ways to care for their health. Scientific research now corroborates what traditional wisdom knew—that medicinal plants can be appropriately and reliably used both to support baseline well-being and treat certain illnesses. While herbal remedies are not meant to replace professional guidance, incorporating them judiciously as a supplement to standard therapies can empower self-care when combined prudently. Herbal medicine continues to emerge as a worthwhile complement to healthcare aimed at preventing issues and strengthening one's natural resilience with Earth's organic, adaptable resources.

Herbalism is regaining prominence as part of mainstream healthcare choices. A sizable portion of people express wanting to try plant-based remedies, seeing them as less processed and potentially safer than manufactured medications. This desire for natural solutions matches broader lifestyle trends embracing organic eating, environmentally friendly practices, and mindfully sourced consumer goods. Global appreciation increases for ancient medical systems like traditional Chinese medicine and Ayurveda, which utilize multi-herb prescriptions. Moreover, the easy access provided by university herbal medicine courses and well-stocked natural health stores' extensive botanical products contributes to reintroducing herbalism as a meaningful option within regular discussions of whole-body wellness approaches.

By blending tried-and-true botanical knowledge with modern production practices and oversight, a vibrant contemporary herbal industry has emerged to meet diverse needs. Some individuals primarily utilize herbalist guidance for healthcare optimization, while others see it as valuable supplementation alongside standard medical support. Herbs can bolster baseline wellness by reinforcing immune function and vitality, as well as address lingering issues like inflammation, anxiety, sleep disturbances, hormonal issues, and minor illnesses with relatively few side effects compared to medications in many cases. For serious health events demanding immediate attention, herbs then play a secondary rather than primary role, working together with mainstream treatments. This integration illustrates how blending diverse perspectives can maximize individualized care, with herbalism's role ranging from stand-alone to collaborative depending on circumstance.

Through applying contemporary investigative tools, science is now corroborating what herbalism's practitioners knew anecdotally for ages: That certain plant-based treatments do indeed exert tangible impacts on our biology. Research identifies which herb extracts and essential oils actively counter microbial overgrowth, oxidative damage, and cancerous spread, both in lab experiments and in living subjects (Herman et al., 2012), (Parham et al., 2020), and (Kaefer and Milner, 2011). Populace analyses also link certain botanical remedies to enhanced immune and metabolic functioning (Khalid et al., 2022). While herbs taken judiciously generally support wellness, integrative medical frameworks help establish standardized dosage advisories and quality benchmarks to help guide safe, efficacious herb use as natural adjuncts. Such research brings empirical confirmation that some inexpensive organic compounds hold real healing properties worth preserving and applying judiciously as a result.

The worldwide scientific community acknowledges traditional herbal medicine as a worthwhile wisdom system to safeguard, maintain, and explore more deeply. After all, the riches of the plant kingdom have already granted people extraordinarily helpful remedies, from foxglove heart management to periwinkle cancer treatments. Yet only a small fraction of Earth's quarter-million higher plant types have undergone examination, indicating further discovery potential in herbs. Researchers propose respectful teamwork with Indigenous communities possessing an intergenerational wealth of botanical insights as one path to more quickly finding novel solutions for new sicknesses facing society (Aziz et al., 2018). By building trust and knowledge-sharing between diverse perspectives, progress could unfold while upholding natural and cultural heritage, highlighting how valuing our shared natural and social diversity strengthens healthcare access globally.

As more people inclusively manage health using various modalities, medical training is properly enhancing herbal education. Doctors, nurses, and other practitioners are also equipped to counsel patients, combining herbal remedies with drug regimens, should they comprehend plants' actions. Most American medical colleges now provide optional herbal medicine classes or incorporate herbal discussions into relevant scientific courses so future providers recognize safe, judicious integration. Some nursing, pharmacy, and nutrition programs also raise awareness of the herb-drug interplay. Evolving healthcare policies are designing frameworks embracing whole-person care, including botanical wisdom tailored for communities' self-care needs. Such adaptations mean all may benefit, whether solely or complementarily, by drawing upon nature's solutions alongside modern approaches.

Moving forward, herbalism stands poised to blend both ancestral plant knowledge and biomedical insights in a truly complementary symphony. As environmental health and human health indelibly intertwine, perhaps rekindling our kinship with plants offers nourishing preventatives and therapeutic synergies we have yet to fully realize. When applied with care and understanding, herbal medicine certainly holds great promise.

Understanding Herbal Actions and Energetics

Herbalism employs plants for healing purposes due to their special mixes of natural compounds interacting purposefully in the human body. Herbs demonstrate particular functions aimed at protecting health or relieving sickness. For example, some support the liver, others ease the pain. Ancient medical systems such as Ayurveda and Traditional Chinese Medicine (TCM) also categorize herbs in terms of energy properties to balance individual constitutional imbalances. By considering an herb's known medicinal roles plus its energetics, herbalists can tailor plant-based therapies that match people's unique circumstances holistically. This personalized matching addresses both symptoms and underlying wellness, demonstrating how harnessing nature's treatments strategically supports whole-being health nourished at the source when needs and attributes come into alignment.

Basics of Herbal Actions

Herbs obtain their special healing properties thanks to arrays of biologically functional elements. For example, some notable anti-inflammatory herbs like turmeric, white willow, and ginger reduce prostaglandins and histamines linked to swelling, aches, and fevers. Immunostimulant plants, including garlic, echinacea, and goldenseal, back up our defenses against bacterial and viral illnesses. Nervine herbs such as oat straw, lavender, and lemon balm possess qualities that precisely contact our nerve pathways, allowing relaxation or activation psychologically as situations require. Beyond these representative examples, diverse herbal actions tonify organs, soothe coughs, regulate menstruation, improve cardiovascular function, enhance cognition, and much more.

Herbal combinations thoughtfully unite plants' functions, magnifying wellness gains. Astragalus and reishi mushrooms, as immunostimulating adaptogens, bolster reserves, defending against wear and tear. Licorice, marshmallow, and slippery elm contain substances that create soothing protective coatings within respiratory and digestive routes vulnerable to harm. Herbal ingredients disperse unequally across our diverse bodily domains when taken internally. Therefore, skillfully correlating specific properties with treatment goals optimizes natural support systems. This nuanced, strategic blending confirms how, considering the complex dance between substances, human attributes, and health situations, herbalism's most expertly nurturing applications harmonize body, mind, and spirit.

Energetics in Herbalism

Expanding beyond biochemical mechanisms, traditional herbalism views vital energy flowing through the body as mediating health versus disease states. This vital force integrates energetic influences embodied in plants to harmonize imbalances. Diagnostic frameworks like Ayurvedic doshas and the Chinese Five Element theory distinguish each person's predominant constitutions and guide which plant energies heal specific deficiencies.

In Ayurveda, the three doshas comprise combinations of *Vata* (air/wind), *Pitta* (fire), and *Kapha* (earth/water) energies both in the body and environment. Ginger carries heating stimulant energy to remedy cold stagnation, whereas rose calms hot inflammatory excess. In TCM, warming *yang* tonics like ginseng treat chilliness and fatigue, while cooling *yin* demulcents like aloe vera reduce inflammatory heat signs. Observing holistic patterns, herbalists cross-culturally prescribe plant synergies to align vital forces within a person with their habitat, community, and metaphysical state.

Beyond categorical actions, close observation reveals how plants communicate deeper sustenance through their very presence in our lives. The interdependent ecology between human health and environmental well-being underlies herbalism's historical endurance. Beholding the beauty of herbs growing wild, appreciating seasonal cycles, preparing remedies, and ingesting whole plant medicines reconnect us with nature's empowering wisdom. We have only begun elucidating the medicinal gems these ancient green friends pass along.

Safety and Efficacy in Herbal Practice

Responsible and ethical use of herbal medicine takes both safety and efficacy seriously. While plants offer therapeutic potential with fewer side effects than pharmaceutical drugs in most cases, mismanaged botanicals can also lead to complications. By learning prudent guidelines, evaluating individual needs, sourcing reputable products, and administering appropriate dosages, herbal remedies boost wellness exceedingly well.

Importance of Safety

Herbal medicine demonstrates an admirable safety record, especially regarding chronic use for optimal health. Therapeutic phytochemicals often mitigate their own toxicity. However, irresponsible formulation, dosage, or contamination can pose problems with anything potent. Certain contraindicated situations also warrant caution when using specific herbs. For example, pregnant women ought to avoid stimulating or detoxifying botanicals but indulge in nutritive herbs like red raspberry leaf safely.

Your personal wellness targets matter when choosing suitable options. Ensuring high quality is key. Proper identification, clean facilities, correct harvest times, safe extraction methods, and lab testing make sure plants are pure—free from toxins or other contaminants. Tailoring preparations with optimal solvents and sterile equipment prevents unwanted extras. Following sensible safety tips significantly reduces risks. Taking these steps respects tradition while adapting knowledge positively. It means natural remedies' benefits can shine through for personalized care. With prudence and progress partnering, herbalism's ancestral strengths serve modern well-being.

Potential problems come primarily from misinformation or dubious products. Jumping in with too-high amounts without checking the impact or lacking clear facts about what you're using could cause undesirable symptoms. For safe choices, it's crucial to get plant identification right—for example, telling foxglove's digitalis from comfrey leaf, which are quite different with opposite effects. Unverified online chatter isn't a smart self-care guide. Reputable texts and trustworthy sources will help you gain a valid understanding to make well-informed decisions. Taking the time to educate yourself protects your health and means natural treatments' successes can truly shine through. With mindful preparation, herbalism's gifts keep flowing for positive well-being.

Above all, herbs serve preventatively for long-term wellness rather than quick fixes that tempt overuse. Habitual low doses enhance function without disrupting homeostasis abruptly. Occasionally pausing to observe subtle shifts allows the body to integrate herbal input before resuming treatment. Holism considers each person's circumstances through in-depth dialogue rather than broad assumptions. Thus, integrating safety into herbal practice honors the ultimate injunction to "first, do no harm."

Evaluating Herbal Efficacy

The potency of herbal medicine hinges significantly on harvested plant quality, preparation methods, and matched dosage for therapeutic purposes. Wild specimens gathered at peak seasons from pristine habitats tend to convey a higher medicinal quality. Combining plants can enhance benefits synergistically. Tinctures in alcohol base the extracts synergistically and preserve for several years, whereas teas or glycerites impart qualities better taken fresh. Culinary spices used daily promote general wellness through diet. Capsules standardized to marker compounds assure potency.

Timing matters too; regular, small amounts deliver persistent support without the system getting used to it. Some herbs offer protective boosts or short mood lifts now and then, as needed. For ongoing concerns, subtle and steady use handles troubles in a balanced way without overpowering nature. Practitioners craft personalized, multi-step plans tailored to the individual. They modify remedies carefully over time to lovingly guide well-being back to its source. True healing means living vibrantly without symptoms, not just masking issues. With nuance and nurturing through phases, ancient wisdom empowers thriving holistically—body and soul.

The efficacy of herbal interventions relies substantially on individualizing preparative elements while regularly reevaluating progress. While plants offer wonderful wellness support, one size does not fit all. Each herb has distinct gifts that need the right preparation—from harvesting to how it's made and taken—to shine in healing. Maximizing these subtle nuances taps ancestral wisdom continually refined through close attention across eras. By drawing on history's insights while adapting individualized plans with care, herbalism's potent yet peaceful legacy endures. Its gifts flow unstopped when shared flexibly yet faithfully between generations. Tradition strengthens through respectful evolution; ancient strengths survive by serving new friends freshly. With patience over time, herbalism's potent yet peaceful legacy endures.

Chapter 2

Getting Started with Herbal Gardening

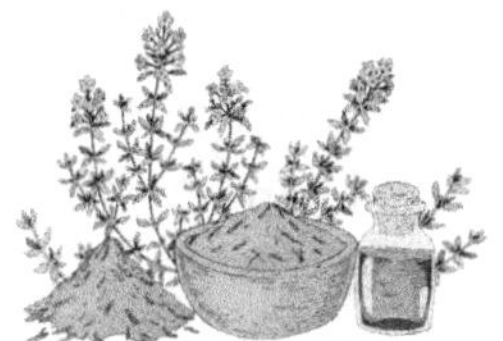

Growing an herbal garden with healing plants you can use for natural remedies offers profoundly nourishing rewards. Through the cultivation of these live botanical partners in your garden, you can access ancient plant knowledge that our ancestors have used for ages to stay well. Your garden will not just beautify your landscape but also impart therapeutic gifts and encourage a connection with the natural cycles of the environment.

As much as it involves our hands, gardening engages our souls as well, allowing us to participate in the green growth that brings healing and hope. Come work in the soil and allow a deep-rooted relationship with medicinal plants.

Choosing Your Medicinal Garden's Location

Selecting an optimal location on your property for cultivating medicinal herbs requires assessing sunlight availability, evaluating soil quality characteristics, or considering container gardening alternatives. Careful planning allows your future garden to thrive sustainably.

Sunlight Requirements

Sun-loving plants like thyme, rosemary, lavender, lemon balm, and sage thrive with at least six hours of direct sunlight daily. Dappled shade under trees is plenty for goldenseal, chives, celery, and echinacea. Nevertheless, most herbs cannot photosynthesize well in order to produce enough energy and biomass when they are in deep shadow. When selecting a site, pay attention to how the patterns of sunlight change with the seasons.

Track sunlight duration in potential garden sites at summer and winter solstices. In the Northern Hemisphere, summertime peak intensity is experienced by south-facing zones during midday. East-facing lands gather gentle morning sun in summer and some afternoon sun in winter. West sides may overheat in summer, but welcome sunset rays in winter. It is common for gradient microclimates to develop inside one terrain. If no evenly sunny exposure exists, consider a succession of smaller beds following sunlight patterns.

As the sun dips lower in the winter, be mindful of nearby structures that may ultimately shadow off certain spots. Avoiding too much shade is ideal when using tall trees that only begin to leaf out in the middle of spring. Additionally, the slope features direct wind and moisture, changing the potential for herb growth. Monitor rainfall-runoff, frost pockets, and drying exposure when assessing microclimates.

Soil Considerations

Most herbs prefer loamy, humus-rich soil with substantial organic matter and moderate drainage capacity. More amendments are needed in dense clay or very sandy soils in order to enhance nutrition, moisture retention, and root aeration. The ideal pH range for mineral availability is 6-7, but some acid-lovers like blueberries thrive at 5 pH, and alkaline-preferring plants like lavender tolerate up to 8 pH.

Simple home soil test kits check pH and macronutrient content to understand baseline needs. Compost, aged manure, peat moss, leaf mold, and grass clippings all increase soil fertility and water-holding capacity. Specific mineral amendments address deficiencies. For example, wood ash raises pH, whereas sulfur reduces alkalinity. Alpine strawberries love calcium; nettles are obsessed with phosphorus. Thus, evaluating soil informs nutrient adjustments for happy herbs.

Container Gardening

For urban gardeners or properties with poor drainage, soil contamination, or unfavorable microclimates, cultivating herbs in containers provides flexibility. Potted plants can move across patios and balconies to maximize sunlight exposure, manipulate moisture levels, and expand planting space creatively in small areas. Self-watering buckets facilitate growth even while traveling. Productive soil mixes for container herbs feature coconut coir or bark, perlite or vermiculite, worm castings, and slow-release organic fertilizer. Just ensure to water sufficiently and renew the soil annually. With the right soil blend, potted herbs yield abundantly.

Understanding Your Climate and Hardiness Zone

Local environmental factors significantly influence herbs' ability to thrive, including rainfall, wind patterns, humidity, seasonal temperature flux, chill hours, and frost dates. Consulting hardiness zone maps further clarifies which plants tolerate your area's winter lows for better selection. Tailoring botanical choices for your garden's unique climate allows medicinal plants to gift their best vitality.

Importance of Climate Awareness

The different types of herbs we grow do best when cared for in conditions similar to where they originally came from in nature. For example, Mediterranean herbs like rosemary, thyme, and oregano are used in mild winters with rain, followed by long, hot, and dry summers. Tropical herbs such as ginger, turmeric, basil, and moringa need warm, humid conditions without frost. Herbs from cooler northern forests like mullein, nettle, and juniper grow well with abundant sunshine and milder summers. Understanding climate cues guides appropriate plant selection, spacing, watering, and fertilization for optimal health.

Pay attention to your location's typical weather from season to season. Notice things like when snow melts in spring, the hottest months of summer, how winds usually blow, and when the first fall frost happens. Certain areas, like low valleys and hills, can experience different conditions. Location matters too; land near coasts, cities, or country areas may have their own microclimates. Take notes on these trends over a few years to best understand your yard's characteristics. This informs garden layout, cold protection tactics, irrigation planning, and whether to amend native soils that sustain local natives. Observing Mother Nature where you live helps your whole garden thrive naturally.

As a resilient precaution against climate unpredictability, it is ideal to cultivate locally native wildcrafted herbs that are biologically suited to your county. But also take into account popular near-native imports that integrate well and have healing benefits. Responsible exotic introductions respectfully honor their heritage through habitat similarities. Thus, climate awareness allows medicinal botanicals to share their gifts sustainably.

Hardiness Zones

Hardiness zone maps can be really helpful planning tools. Developed from long-term weather tracking, they divide the world into numbered zones based on typical winter low temperatures, from the coldest Zone 1 areas to the warmest Zone 11 regions. Plant tags also list a range of compatible zones. By checking your zone on the map, you can get an idea if a tempting new plant like a Japanese maple or cactus could handle your area's coldest winters or hottest summers before deciding to grow it. The maps take the guesswork out of whether plants that caught your eye might struggle where you live.

Consult reliable zone maps to cross-reference with herb descriptions for projected overwintering capacity and harvest longevity. For example, echinacea thrives in Zones 3–10, whereas bushy Mexican oregano suits hot, arid Zones 8–11. Knowing your zone along with microclimate nuances prevents plants from succumbing to colds that outstrip their resilience. It also guides cold protection measures like mulching for border-line hardy herbs.

Since zones identify survivability rather than productivity thresholds, certain plants stretch beyond their ideal vigor range if sheltered during temperature extremes. Experiment to determine whether a cherished plant that would usually be rated for nearby zones may adorn your landscape wonderfully with some assistance. Climate change also alters the applicability of dated zones over time. However, hardiness zones provide useful advice to guarantee that the medicinal plants entrusted to your care can continue to work their therapeutic magic for many years to come.

Selecting Herbs for Your Garden

Stock your budding medicinal garden with reliable, easy-care herbs along with personalized picks to suit your wellness goals. Planting companion plants strategically enables friends to organically support one another. Crafting a thoughtful custom herbal sanctuary will reward you richly for years as your refuge and pharmacy.

Medicinal Herbs for Beginners

When starting your first healing garden, focus on resilient, prolific herbs that thrive readily in your climate. These hardy yet generous beauties provide plenty of medicinal flowers, leaves, roots, and seeds while also assisting new gardeners in gaining confidence. Favored starter herbs include calendula, chamomile, parsley, sage, thyme, lemon balm, peppermint, echinacea, and valerian.

Lettuce leaf basil, dill, bee balm, yarrow, and elderberry also prosper easily. Garlic, onion, shallot, and sorrel serve up edible medicine from the lily family. Fast-spreading kitchen staples like oregano, rosemary, and mint generously provide taste and health benefits. This medley of starter herbs presents diverse wellness properties like anti-inflammatory, antimicrobial, pain-relieving, digestive-enhancing, and anxiety-reducing actions.

Personalizing Your Garden

After you've grown a few core herbal allies, concentrate your next garden additions on your own health objectives. Mullein, coltsfoot, horehound, and licorice roots support lung strength for respiratory problems. Chamomile, marshmallow, aloe vera, and bupleurum are digestive herbs that soothe upset stomachs. Additionally, the vast herbal arsenal improves blood circulation, lymphatic function, hormone balance, blood sugar regulation, heart health, immunity, pain reduction, inflammation reduction, oxidation prevention, pathogen restriction, and exceptionally good toxicity mitigation. Establish priorities before purposefully filling the beds.

Also, intersperse some beautiful flowering options purely for your soul, like sunflowers, nasturtiums, and passionflowers, to ensure joy thrives in your sanctuary. This boutique asylum grows with you over time, becoming a caring green pharmacy that welcomes you home to healing, all according to your unique constitution.

Companion Planting

Certain medicinal botanicals flourish near specific plant partners that enhance nutrition uptake, repel pests, or attract pollinators through symbiotic root exchanges and aromatic synergies. For example, pairing thyme with cabbage deters destructive moths. Tall sunflowers shelter lettuce and bush beans and help strawberries thrive. Dill, cilantro, and chervil grow wonderfully together. Prudent botany pairings promote reciprocal flourishing.

Some combinations even increase medical strength; for example, garlic protects roses against insects while boosting the antibacterial properties of flowers. To ensure that taller friends don't shadow out lower-lying plants, more observation is necessary. Gardens become considerably more resilient ecologies when thoughtful planting strategies based on natural plant friendships are implemented. As a result, companion planting enables your healing haven to develop into an independent permaculture gem that offers you healing sustenance.

Tools of the Trade

Equipping an herbal gardener's toolbox allows efficient, enjoyable cultivation for abundant medicinal harvests. Core instruments like trowels, pruners, and tilling forks ease digging, weeding, and harvesting. Specialty tools facilitate the preparation of herbal products. Organic fertilizers amend soil nutrition deficiencies so herbs thrive. Responsible watering hydrates plants while conserving resources. Investing in quality implements and infrastructure makes steadfast garden stewardship a pleasure.

Essential Gardening Tools

Basic digging tools like round-tip trowels, long-handled cyst forks, ergonomic rakes, and digging shovels facilitate turning soil, smoothing beds, dividing roots, and transferring bulbs with minimal strain. Bypass pruners snip stems cleanly; Hori Hori knives dig deep or saw roots. Watering cans with removable roses gently saturate seedlings. Sturdy but lightweight wheelbarrows transport loads efficiently.

Dedicated herb snips, such as parsley or fennel, make harvesting certain herbs easier without bruising the leaves. Garnishes for bouquets are evenly clipped using garden scissors. A yard of burlap bags keeps drying leaves intact for processing. Herbal medicines should be stored in sterilized ball jars. Kitchen herb racks are a great way to keep fresh herbs like dill or basil vibrant. Thus, purpose-specific instruments optimize efficiency.

Electric tillers and chipper-shredders, in addition to manual analog equipment, expedite bed preparation and cleanup when hand tools strain muscles. High-quality, sharp instruments, such as tempered forged steel blades, save you money and the earth's mines from needless replacement. Long-lasting craftsmanship is more respectful to future generations than disposable items, which devalue the environment.

Soil Amendments and Fertilizers

Organic fertilizer options like aged manure, leaf compost, grass clippings, eggshells, or seed meals slowly release nutrients, improving moisture retention and microbial balances that break down minerals for better plant uptake. Cover crops such as legumes, buckwheat, and alfalfa also improve the nitrogen content and sequester carbon, enriching herb health.

Specific soil deficiencies show up in certain symptom patterns. Yellowing leaves reveal a nitrogen shortage; rust spots on leaves indicate an iron shortage. Wood ash adds potassium and calcium; bone and blood meals boost phosphorus. Thus, targeted amendments counter characteristic deficits.

Watering Strategies

Herbs grow best when there is consistent moisture throughout the root zone and then a period of drying out in between waterings. Most need one to two inches of water each week from irrigation or rain. Instead of using sprinklers, which encourage foliar fungus, soaker hoses, drip irrigation, and water spikes concentrate moisture toward plant stems. Digital moisture meter probes are useful for estimating the next watering time.

Rainfall collected in barrels or cisterns provides naturally gentle precipitation and reduces the need for municipal sources. Rain gardens enable the soil to absorb excess water, while bioswales stop runoff erosion. Applying water consciously utilizes this precious shared resource responsibly. Thus, appropriate tools and infrastructure boost herb cultivation and conservation efforts for bountiful, sustainable gardens.

Maintenance and Care

Regular care for medicinal plants creates robust, healthy gardens. Careful observation identifies when plant demands are expressed by identifying pests, drought stress, or nutrient shortages. Herbs are then carefully cultivated through customized treatments to achieve maximum well-being. Every botanical personality may thrive when a consistent routine of careful attention, accurate pruning, defensive shielding, and preventative care is established.

Regular Care Routine

Herbs thrive on routine care attuned to their natural patterns. Regular, gentle trimming back of leafy growth encourages bushy plants like basil, lemon balm, marjoram, and rosemary. Thinning congested young seedlings allow adequate air circulation, which reduces fungal infections. Mulching and weeding keep moisture levels up, prevent weeds from stifling plants, and restore nutrients as materials decompose.

Examining the undersides of leaves exposes small insects such as Japanese beetles chewing holes or sap-sucking aphids. Stop infestations before they become colonies. Remove pests manually, spray them off with water, or apply gentle insecticidal soap sparingly. Keep an eye out for symptoms of excessive air moisture, such as powdery mildew, black spots, or blight. To prevent spreading, increase ventilation and solar exposure while quickly eliminating contaminated areas.

Certain plants require specific seasonal care. Motherwort, skullcap, and rosemary all flourish when sometimes trimmed in the summertime. In some regions, evergreen Mediterranean woody plants like rosemary need to be protected from severe winter cold. Every year, observe plant indications to comprehend their specific wants.

Pruning and Harvesting Guidelines

Cutting half of the younger top growth of most leafy annual herbs encourages branching, which greatly boosts harvests. Prudent pruning encourages regrowth without putting plants under undue stress. Remember not to shear more than 30% of the leaves at once. The best times to pick herbs are in the early morning, just after the dew has evaporated, or before the flowers open when their medicinal chemistry is at its peak. Know each plant's peak potency season.

When enjoying flowers in nature, leave some behind for helpful bugs like bees and butterflies. This feeds wild animals and spreads diversity. Watching plant seeds ripen tells you the right time to collect and save seeds from plants adapted to your area. These seeds will pass on genetic strengths. If you gather extras, scatter them back where the plants grew. This keeps wildflower patches alive and thriving for years to come. By caring for nature's gifts, you help wildlife and the landscape around us both now and tomorrow.

If we pay close attention to our healing plants throughout the seasons, watching how each one grows and changes, our gardens will thrive. Making time to understand an herb's unique needs, lifecycle patterns, and habitat health allows these wonderful plants to share their gifts like nourishment, lovely sights, and peaceful spaces. With gentle, regular care, an expert bond grows between gardeners and nature's wisdom. Gardens always reward kindness with abundance.

Chapter 3

Soil and Compost Mastery

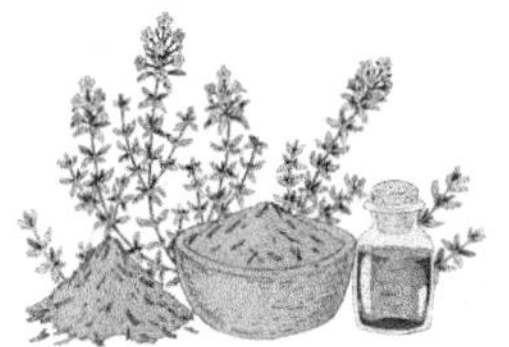

The very ground below is the key to a flourishing garden. The soil is alive with tiny helpers like bacteria, fungi, and earthworms. It holds precious minerals that feed our plants. When the soil is rich and full of life, the plants can thrive and share their goodness with us. Making compost, or recycled plant matter and food scraps, replenishes the soil. This allows more of those mini helpers to dwell there. By learning about soil and building its fertility, we lay the foundation for an abundant garden.

Knowing the science behind composting and soil ecology helps us to better appreciate nature's amazing cycles of decomposition and regeneration. The priceless material that gives us our foundation also feeds the plants that provide us with sustenance, nourishment, and healing. Working hand in hand with the dark alchemy of decomposition that runs the world, we complete a fundamental circuit by collecting health from plants grown in our enhanced soil.

The Life Within the Soil

In the soil live many tiny creatures like bacteria, fungi, and worms that all work together to keep the soil healthy. They break down dead material so nutrients can feed plants. Fungi help plants get water and minerals. Worms and bugs mix everything up and keep air in the soil. When these little helpers are happy, the plants thrive. Taking care of the soil means taking care of all the microbes and organisms below ground. Healthy soil means healthy plants above ground. With the right conditions underground, your garden will be full of lush, vibrant growth. Understanding this interconnected web and cultivating beneficial soil life bolsters above-ground health.

Soil Microorganisms

Numerous single-celled bacteria, actinomycetes, cyanobacteria, algae, and protozoa found in soil are incredibly diverse and drive important chemical processes that prepare fundamental elements that plant cells can absorb and use for sustenance. Different types break down nutrients locked in rocks and make them soluble in water, so plants can use them. Some take nitrogen from the air and fix it into the soil, so plants have this essential element. Others help decompose dead material like leaves to turn them back into nutrients. As they go about these jobs, they protect plants from diseases too.

The helpful microbes cluster around plant roots because the roots release sugar, proteins, and acids. This is like a little reward for the microbes. In return, they provide minerals and special substances that help roots grow bigger and protect against diseases. Some microbes even live right inside plant tissues. We can encourage lots of different microbes and help them thrive by watering with compost tea, planting cover crops to feed the soil, and disturbing the soil less with tilling. This makes the soil and plants healthier at the same time. A variety of soil microbes is like an insurance policy; the more kinds there are, the better they can support plant growth and keep diseases away.

Soil Food Web

Dr. Elaine Ingham discovered that the soil food web concept illuminates a whole interconnected living system, from the smallest microbes, too tiny to see, up to bigger creatures like bugs and worms (Hawk, 2022). All sorts of different organisms break down dead material, convert it into nutrients that plants can use, and support each other in the process. It's like a complex food chain underground. Bacteria provide a food source for tiny nematode worms. Single-celled protozoa eat nitrogen-fixing bacteria to help regulate their numbers. Fungi even capture some nematodes to keep everything in balance. As each member plays their role, they improve the soil. If one piece is missing, it affects the whole web. Understanding these relationships gives us insight into how to nurture a diverse community of soil life.

As all the tiny underground creatures work together to break things down, important nutrients like nitrogen, phosphorus, potassium, and micronutrients become available for plant roots to take up. At the same time, the life teeming within fills the soil with small air pockets and crevices between particles where roots might develop. The intricate hidden world nourishes what we see on top. Understanding this amazing underground network explains how vibrant plant growth is possible. Realizing how dependent the plants are on the complex soil community should inspire us to care for the whole system, not just the greens we see, by nurturing the diversity of life beneath the surface.

Soil Types and Amendments

Building rich, well-structured soil that is compatible with the local geology and enhanced with organic matter through specific amendments is essential to growing vibrant medicinal plants. Finding out the texture, drainage capacity, and nutritional profile of your natural soil enables tailored improvement for successful herbal gardening. Carefully applying mulch preserves moisture, suppresses weed growth, and enhances soil biology.

Overview of Soil Types

Major soil kinds are categorized based on the relative amounts of sand, silt, and clay particles. These types of soil have different characteristics. More than half of the sand grains in sandy soils are bigger, which improves drainage and aeration but reduces water and nutrient retention. Soils with more silt are better at retaining moisture. Clay soils with more than 40% fine clay particles absorb even higher water volumes but often compact poorly drained dense masses. The majority of garden soils are loams, which combine clay, silt, and sand in certain proportions to provide moderate fertility and drainage.

If you dig up soil from different spots, even within your yard, you may notice variations. Nutrient amounts, acidity levels, and saltiness change from place to place too. While a trustworthy lab analysis helps determine demands, basic texture tests work very well as well. When clay is damp, it clusters together and shears quickly when pinched. Sandy grit lacks cohesion, wet or dry. Loamy silt crumbles loosely when dry and blends malleably wet. Knowing the type determines which amendments to focus on, like compost for clay or sand, since plants prefer specific fertility and water-holding abilities. Matching amendments to soil types sets up herbs and gardens for optimal growing conditions.

Soil Amendments

Soil amendments change the texture to get the loamier balance between clay, sand, and silt. This loamy blend suits most plants. Amendments also replace nutrients that herbs need to grow their best but may be missing, like nitrogen for leaves, phosphorus for roots and buds, and potassium for chemical processes inside the plant. Calcium helps plants take up water and nutrients too. Zinc and boron are important for flowering. With the right amendments tailored to your soil, herbs will be healthier and more productive because their basic needs and the ecosystem in the dirt are supported.

Organic compost, aged animal manures, green cover crop plow-under, forest duff layers, dried blood and bone meals, and trace mineral mixes all slowly break down over time and provide herbs with important nutrients. Drainage is also key; the soil needs to allow air and water to move through it easily so plant roots and microbes can thrive. By balancing the soil's content, structure, and microscopic life in organic amendments, your herbs will flourish. Focus on adding materials like compost or manure to feed the soil food web while ensuring excess water can drain out freely.

When preparing garden beds for herbs, be generous with compost. Spreading a thin layer one to three inches thick, or mixing some into the soil around new plants, provides a feast for the microorganisms and earthworms in the soil. As they break down the organic matter, nutrients become available for herbal growth. Other all-natural amendments like well-rotted manure, alfalfa meal, seaweed, fish bones, eggshells, and wood ash sustainably enrich the earth. Herbs and unseen soil life form a symbiotic relationship; as the microbes' health improves with nutrient-dense food sources, so too does the development and flavor of your herbs.

Mulching for Soil Health

When growing herbs, using mulch on the soil surface offers many benefits. Materials like leaves, straw, wood chips, or gravel help regulate moisture loss from the ground and protect roots from extreme heat or cold. As the mulch layers decompose, they replenish the earth's nutrients too. Finely shredded leaves mix readily into the soil. Larger wood chips from trees break down slowly, feeding soil life for many seasons. Gravel prevents erosion. Even black plastic can aid heat retention. The best herb gardens utilize various mulches tailored for drainage and environmental conditions, cultivating healthy, balanced soil ecosystems and maximizing the growth of medicinal plants.

When designing an herbal garden, taking cues from native woodland habitats provides multiple benefits. Certain plants have evolved to thrive together naturally. For instance, mushrooms help break down fallen leaves and branches under the shade of wild plants like black cohosh and mayapple. Pine needles create acidic soil perfectly suited to wild ginger root and partridgeberry. By mimicking these native ecosystems with your own amendments or mulches, both the soil and herbs enjoy balanced growth. They form mutually supportive relationships underground. Paying close attention to cultivating conditions at the roots empowers the plants to grow abundantly.

Building and Maintaining a Compost Pile

Making your own compost is a great way to reuse everyday items and natural waste products to support your herbal garden. Through composting, food scraps, yard trimmings, and manure break down into a nutrient-rich soil amendment called "humus." With a little know-how about keeping the materials moist and evenly mixed, you'll have nutrient-packed compost in no time. Even small spaces are suitable for composting. The environmental and gardening benefits are huge; your herbs will thrive with this organic boost while less gets thrown away. Composting is truly a natural, circular solution that's good for both the planet and your homegrown medicine chest.

Basics of Composting

Making compost is a sustainable way to reuse organic materials instead of throwing them out. The process relies on nature's principles to break everything down into valuable fertilizer. By alternating green, nitrogen-rich ingredients like food scraps with brown, carbon-based ones like shredded leaves in your compost pile, you set up the right conditions for microbes to do their work. As the microbes break down the layers, the inside of the pile heats up on its own. Turning the pile periodically introduces airflow to help the breakdown progress evenly. In a matter of months, your pile is transformed into crushed compost—nutrient-packed soil food for your herbs.

When building a compost pile, include both green and brown ingredients for balance. Green items provide nitrogen in the form of nitrogen-rich foods and plant materials like grass clippings, fresh weeds, coffee grounds, manure, and fruit and vegetable scraps. Browns are carbon sources like dried leaves, sawdust, and straw. Aim to use one part green to three parts brown materials (Vanderlinden, 2009). This carbon-nitrogen ratio gives the microbes the right ratio of fuel to feed on. Avoid meat, oils, or fatty foods, which can attract pests. Stick to about 30% greens by volume to support the bustling microbe population, breaking everything down into rich compost for your garden.

When building a compost pile, be sure to include brown materials high in carbon, like dried leaves, straw, sawdust, or shredded paper. These act as a slow-release energy source for microbes as well as help regulate moisture levels. Other options are items such as dried grass, corn stalks, small wood chips, hay, nut shells, or pine needles. Layering different browns and greens creates air pockets through the pile. Be sure to turn the compost every month or so if using a pile or container, or every 2-3 months if in a longer window. This stirs things up and spreads the microbes, nutrients, and moisture evenly for faster breakdown. You'll know the compost is ready when it has an earthy smell, feels damp but not soggy, and crumbles easily—perfectly rich soil for nourishing herbs and plants.

Troubleshooting Common Composting Issues

If your compost pile isn't breaking down properly, some simple adjustments may help. Bad smells usually mean too much green material, too much moisture trapped inside, or not enough airflow. To remedy this, add more dried leaves, wood chips, or other browns to soak up extra liquid and balance the carbon-to-nitrogen ratio. Be sure to turn the pile every month or so to introduce oxygen pockets as it breaks down. You can also use a long PVC pipe or hollow rebar to create tunnels through the pile. Wood ash helps neutralize odors by raising the pH to a healthier level for microbes. With a little experimenting, you'll troubleshoot composting in no time to yield rich soil for your garden.

If your compost seems to be breaking down slowly, it may need a nitrogen boost. Steep some comfrey leaves, alfalfa meal, or even coffee grounds in water, then pour the tea onto the pile to feed the microbes. Other excellent green amendments are fresh grass clippings, manure, or cover crops containing legumes. These nitrogen powerhouses will get things heating up again. Be sure the moisture level is barely damp, like a squeezed-out sponge—not bone dry or overly soggy. A tarp over the pile can help hold moisture if it dries out too much.

Whether you have a large yard or just a small balcony, composting is possible with a little creativity. In tighter spaces, just make smaller, more frequent batches that finish quicker. Enclosed bins deter rodents without using pesticides. Look for warm spots too, like where the house meets the ground; compost heats up faster there. And worms are amazing recyclers! Vermicompost bins use red wrigglers to break down scraps inside without smelling. There are composting solutions for every situation, from apartments to acreage. No matter the size of your garden, you can harness nature's process to turn waste into rich, organic fertilizer.

pH and Soil Health

The acidity, or pH, of garden soil, is really important for herbs to grow their best. Most plants like conditions that are mildly acidic to neutral, with a pH between 6.0 and 7.0. If the soil is too far above or below this range, nutrients may not be available to the herbs. Testing soil pH gives you a good idea of how acidic or alkaline it is. From there, small adjustments can be made by adding amendments tailored to individual plant needs. For example, sulfur lowers pH while limestone raises it. Taking pH into account ensures your soil supports optimal herb growth and development.

Importance of pH in Gardening

The pH scale measures how acidic or alkaline the soil is. It runs from 0 to 14, with 7 being neutral. Most plants, including herbs, prefer the mildly acidic range of 6.2–6.7 because nutrient availability is optimal. At low pH, certain minerals like iron are easily absorbed, but phosphate decreases. When soil pH rises above 7.5 into alkaline territory, the opposite happens: Phosphate is plentiful, but iron becomes scarce. The varying pH levels change the chemical forms of nutrients in the earth. This affects which ones the plant roots can take in to nourish growth. Testing and adjusting pH optimizes the soil conditions to ensure herbs get the minerals they need.

The natural pH of the soil is greatly influenced by its parent geological material. Different types of soil—sandy, silty, or clay-based—have pH tendencies reflecting the minerals in the underlying bedrock they formed over thousands of years. However, other factors influence soil pH too, like local rainfall, microbes living in it, and what fertilizers are used. All can make the soil more acidic or alkaline over time. You can test pH easily with an inexpensive home kit. Then balance it as needed for your herbs by adding amendments—things like peat moss or sulfur will lower the pH, while limestone or oyster shell will raise it.

When preparing your herb garden beds, it pays to group plants together that prefer similar soil pH levels. This lets you target amendments for several herbs at a time. For instance, marjoram, lemon balm, chamomile, and basil all thrive when the soil is mildly alkaline, around a pH of 6.7. By adding lime to just one section, you satisfy what all those plants need with one application. Organizing beds based on the pH needs of the herbs makes adjusting the soil much more efficient. Instead of tweaking small areas individually, you take care of whole sections at once. It saves time, effort, and resources to understand pH requirements and plan plant communities accordingly.

pH Preferences of Medicinal Herbs

When setting up your medicinal herb garden, it's helpful to know the best pH ranges for different groups. Many popular culinary herbs like mint, oregano, and garlic prefer the mildly acidic 6.0–6.5 level. Sage, rosemary, and thyme also grow well in this slightly acidic soil. Herbs that do well at a near-neutral pH of 6.8–7.0 include parsley, cilantro, dill, and fennel. Lemon balm, chamomile, and calendula tolerate slightly more alkaline conditions up to 7.2, as do moisture-loving herbs like ginger.

However, some medicinal herbs require more acidic or alkaline soil to really flourish. Strawberry plants, blueberry, huckleberry, rhododendrons, azalea, and magnolias need quite acidic ground from pH 5.0–5.5 to take up iron and nutrients, allowing their bright pigments and flavors to shine. Woodland botanicals like goldenseal, black cohosh, and ginseng also relish a pH of around 5.5, close to native deciduous forest floor acidity.

Certain herbs actually prefer more alkaline soil than the normally recommended range. Horehound, soapwort, and yarrow thrive when the pH is between 7.5 and 8.0. Some weeds like dandelion, nettle, and mustard greens also grow well above 7 pH. By accounting for each plant's preferred soil acidity or alkalinity levels, you can amend your beds accordingly to give them their ideal environment. With a bit of pH testing and natural adjustments using materials like compost or lime, you can steward the earth and its microbial life to cultivate mighty, therapeutic herbs in harmony with their needs.

Practical Applications

Now you get to directly apply soil improvement strategies customized to the distinct characteristics of your own garden. With soil testing illuminating native fertility profiles, pH inclination, and texture attributes, you can craft a targeted amendment regimen using compost, organic fertilizers, and pH adjusters to create optimal growing conditions for thriving herbs tailored to your site's unique ecology.

Implementing Soil Amendments Based on Soil Tests

Begin stewarding your medicinal garden by collecting soil samples from multiple areas around your yard or beds to receive a laboratory analysis detailing soil composition. Soil tests measure texture percentages of sand, silt, and clay that determine drainage capacity and nutrient retention alongside fertility indicators of critical elements: Nitrogen for foliage growth, phosphorus for flowering and fruiting, potassium for plant metabolism, calcium, magnesium, and micronutrients like iron, manganese, boron, and zinc. The report will also reveal pH, organic matter content, cation exchange capacity, and levels of certain contaminants if present.

With this baseline data clarifying exactly what your native soil lacks, appropriate amendments become evident. To shift sandier soils toward loamy textures, mix in clay-based topsoil or silt-rich compost to balance texture. Very dense clay blends lighten considerably with additions of aged manure, coir, hay, and shredded autumn leaves to elevate fertility and permeability. Target ideal organic matter. Specific micronutrient deficiencies also emerge for correction—perhaps calcium sulfate for alkalinity or iron phosphate for acid lovers.

Having prepared fertile loam integrating organic compost, cover crop plow-under, and targeted mineral adjustments, group herbs by preferred pH range as you allocate garden beds. Limestone raises the pH of alkaline-loving mints; azaleas need acidic peat conditions. With thoughtful amendments, dirt transforms into living soil where herbs thrive.

Creating a Customized Composting Plan

Grasp opportunities to recycle onsite nutrients by establishing a customized composting system based on available raw materials. Figure out the best setup based on how much organic waste your home produces, like kitchen scraps or garden trimmings. Consider if you'll have lots of leaves, grass clippings, or animal manure too. Those things help determine the size and type of composting method that works best. For example, regular coffee drinkers making tons of garden debris might go for a 3-bin system to handle it all. Balconies and patios are better with enclosed bins to keep things tidy and small enough for regular turning. No matter the space, smart composting lets you recycle nutrients right where they're generated.

Determine your average carbon-to-nitrogen ratio so that extra brown materials, such as sawdust or shredded paper, may be added to balance out excess green material as needed. Track biological activity by keeping an eye on interior temperatures. Then, turn heaps to disperse moisture and nutrients toward the ultimate product—a pathogen-free humus that resembles crumbs from a dark chocolate cake—the best organic fertility additions. Mix the completed compost into each bed and planting hole to provide a base-level nutrient infusion. This will awaken the full fertility of the garden from below.

Monitoring and Adjusting pH as Needed

It's a good idea to check your soil's pH annually since it can fluctuate over time. Heavy rain may make the soil more acidic through leaching. And compost pH shifts seasonally too. If you grow plants that demand a specific pH level, test those beds annually to keep the minerals balanced for optimal growth. Rotating crops with things like legumes, veggies, and flowers also affects pH gradually. Customized amendments tailored to problem spots go a long way too. A bit of sulfur, limestone, or biochar can make areas resistant to change. Small yearly pH adjustments keep your herb gardens and mineral ingredients in top form.

A balanced program nourishes the all-important microbial life, structure, and nutrients that support plant growth. By monitoring soil properties, you can purposefully improve fertility through natural amendments tailored to your specific needs. Working together with nature's conditions and chosen plantings, a little loving care encourages the soil to reach its full abundance-creating potential. Nurturing the earth's living ecosystems lets land heal itself through seasonal cycles of planting and harvest. Healthy soil is the real miracle-maker; it's the foundation that allows any seeds we scatter to truly flourish.

Chapter 4

Propagation Techniques for Medicinal Plants

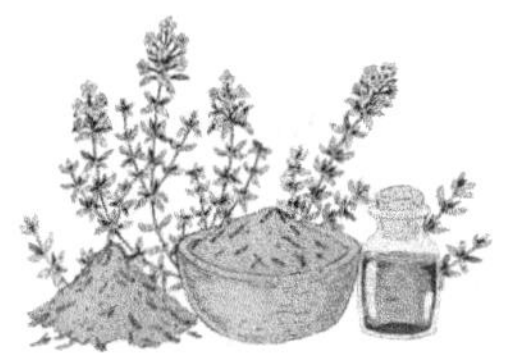

Now that you've put in the effort to build up nutrient-rich, living soil just right for herbs, it's time to introduce some plant friends. You can propagate your favorite medicinal plants in various ways, like seeds, cuttings, dividing established plants, or transplantation. Figure out the best method for each species to encourage robust growth. Nurture the newcomers as they develop their roots. Before you know it, you'll be easily multiplying your most treasured herbs to enjoy yourself and share with community members and other gardeners.

Propagating plants is a really rewarding part of gardening that allows you to connect with nature's incredible regenerative forces up close. Whether starting from seeds, rooting stem cuttings, or transplanting nursery-grown starts, helping herbs multiply touches our soul. It takes a gentle touch and the willingness to watch and wait as new life takes root. Through the simple act of propagation, we support our treasured medicinal plants in reproducing robustly and true to their kind. By cultivating new seedlings, cuttings, or divisions with care and patience, we tap into the profound creative energy inherent in all living things.

Seed Starting Basics

Propagating herbs from seeds connects us to ancient healing traditions stretching back millennia. Those first herbalists recognized plants' amazing abilities and gave us traditions we still rely on. When we grow new generations of medicinal herbs from seeds, we carry on that learning. To be good stewards of that age-old wisdom passed down within seeds, find trustworthy sources and tend seedlings with attentiveness. Things like soil, containers, sunlight, and temperature all affect sprouting success. Addressing any issues ensures healthy growth. Nurturing seeds through their beginnings instills hope and responsibility in gardeners.

Selecting High-Quality Seeds

For the most robust herb seedlings, start with high-quality seeds from reliable sources. Look for organic, non-gmo varieties specializing in medicinal plants. Heirloom and native options do especially well locally. Regional seed swaps offer hardy gems too. Research each tiny treasure since herb seeds have wildly different needs—some keep longer or sprout pickier than others. Plump, smooth, heavy seeds tend to sprout better than shriveled, damaged, or fungus-y ones. Hard shells on seeds protect against aging, while softer kinds can lose sprouting power within a couple years unless refrigerated right with desiccants.

With seeds, it pays to choose varieties with a proven track record that have stood the test of time. Heirloom seeds from open-pollinated, non-hybrid plants retain valuable traits nurtured by generations of selective growing. They uphold suitability, potency, and resilience specifically for your area. Patented sources without background information are less reliable. While hybrids ensure consistent production, the offspring may differ, which is not ideal if you want to save seeds. Heirlooms guarantee reliable reproduction over years. When perpetuating treasured herbs, they can't be beat. Seek out heritage strains developed through centuries of observant ancestral growers—perfected not just by science but by the wisdom of nature and Indigenous communities.

Indoor vs. Outdoor Seed Starting

Starting seeds indoors has advantages: You can keep a close eye on conditions and shield young plants from problems outside like fungi, temperature fluctuations, wind, or slugs. Steering clear of issues like damping off disease gives seedlings a healthy head start. Once they're sturdier, ease transplants outside gradually to adjust. But some herbs don't like their roots disturbed. They do better planted directly where they'll grow rather than being moved twice. So, choose your propagation method thoughtfully, depending on the type of herb. A watchful indoor start or protected direct sowing—both can work well depending on the plant's preferences.

When planting herb seeds outside, timing is key. Pay attention to each plant's preferred soil temperature for sprouting. Some herbs, like cilantro and dill, can handle light frost but don't like summer's heat. Sow them early. Others, such as basil, borage, and calendula, germinate best in warm, loamy soil perfect for planting a bit later. Follow packet directions for specifics on light, moisture, and any unique pre-treatment needs like scratching or chilling seeds. Aim to start so your plants have a full growing season and peak potency near harvest in the fall.

With the right timing aligned with each herb's temperature preferences, you set your seedlings up for success from the very beginning.

Seed Starting Materials and Containers

Big pots can keep the soil too wet and cold, slowing growth. Look for a sterile, fast-draining seed starting mix in the potting medium; it should be light and fluffy to promote tender roots without fungus. Ingredients like vermiculite, peat, or coconut coir provide excellent draining properties, along with a natural fertilizer that won't burn delicate seeds. Steer clear of using garden soil, which may harbor issues or compact heavily. Always clean pots with a 10% bleach solution before reusing them.

Germination Tips

To get herbs growing from seed, start by warming up the soil and moistening it well. Then follow the seed packet instructions to plant at the right depth; bigger seeds go in deeper than smaller ones. Cover the pots or seeds with a plastic dome to keep the moisture up until you see sprouts. As soon as you spot them, take the dome off so the seedlings don't stretch too much, seeking the light. At first, the seed leaves will feed the baby plants until their true leaves emerge. Then you can start giving them diluted fertilizer. Be sure the little plants get enough fresh air flowing so they don't get sick from soil fungus. By sowing certain herbs like cilantro, chervil and salad greens in batches, you can harvest them all season long. Before long, your trays will be full of beautiful green plants, nourishing both your garden and your soul with their progress from seed to leaf!

Vegetative Propagation: Cuttings, Layering, and Division

You can make more copies of your favorite herbs quickly without waiting for seeds by cloning existing plants through simple techniques like cutting, layering, or dividing. Cloning produces exact replicas that share the same resilient traits as the parent. Taking stem or root cuttings while still attached gives the new growth a head start by letting it establish protected roots. Once independent roots have formed, severing the cuttings creates miniature versions ready to thrive on their own. With practice, anyone can multiply their medicinal herb supply endlessly through gentle propagation methods. Mastering these organic arts through thoughtful timing and care transforms single, cherished plants into expansive, healing botanical abundance.

Propagation by Cuttings

Many herbs, both perennial and annual, can be easily multiplied through stem or root cuttings taken from parent plants. Look for specimens that display good characteristics you want to pass on, like potency, hardiness, or productivity. Shrubs and perennials are often rooted in stem pieces, while some annuals prefer root divisions. No matter the type, the secret is to use clean, sharp pruners sterilized with rubbing alcohol to make clean cuts. Snip off pieces when plants are vigorously growing, just before flowering, when nutrients move down to support new roots. These times of active hormones and sugar flow encourage rooted clones to form quickly. By selecting prime parent stock and catching them at their peak seasonal rhythm, plant propagation through cuttings makes it simple to share favorite herbs with fellow gardeners.

For stem cuttings, select non-flowering green stems that are 4-6 inches long, taken from leaf joints rather than woody areas. Trim off lower leaves and use a sharp blade to notch just under bud sites, where roots may develop. Some herbs, such as mint, yarrow, and lavender, only multiply this way. After cutting, dip the bare stems in rooting hormone powder to aid new root growth. Place under a clear plastic dome, which keeps things clean and moist as roots form. Cuttings need plenty of indirect sunlight to make food and grow, but avoid direct sunlight, as it can dry them out. With the right timing, harvesting of parent material, and consistent care, cuttings will take root and leaf out, giving you a bounty of new plants produced naturally from your favorite herbs.

Certain woody plants, such as magnolia, willow, and poplar, are very capable of self-pollination through rhizomes, lateral roots, and prunings that contain bark and wood. These hearty hardwood cuttings are more durable and take to rooting, especially for trees that are difficult to grow from stem pieces. But while rooting occurs quickly, it takes woody clones longer to develop a strong base and put up new leaves and growth— sometimes 1-3 years of waiting patiently. Once established though, they are ruggedly resilient, filling gardens with rapidly spreading colonies of the same desirable plant for generations.

Layering Techniques

An easy way to help cloned herbs and shrubs get a strong foothold is to let stem or root cuttings remain partially connected to the mother plant at first. By leaving them lightly attached rather than fully removed, the parent continues providing water and nutrients through its vascular system until the new growth forms its own root structure. This time-tested layering method gives offspring a boost so they will thrive once on their own two feet. Under the mother's gentle guidance, lateral stems and branches are encouraged to put down adventurous exploratory roots well before full separation once leaves proudly emerge. With this patient approach, cuttings integrate smoothly into independent, but not lone, little versions of beloved parent plants.

There are handy techniques to propagate herbs by layering. Essentially, you bend a flexible stem to lie along a supportive surface, so the point where it touches develops roots while still attached to the parent plant. This could involve gently mounding soil or moss over a portion or weighting sections down with pins until roots form where buried nodes contact the medium. Air layering is similar: Remove a band of bark, wrap damp moss plus rooting hormone powder around the exposed area, and cover it with plastic. Soon new growth occurs, and once fully rooted, you transplant the self-sufficient young plant. This rejuvenates old stock by stimulating youthful new roots, shoots, and productivity without disturbing the established parent herb.

As layered stems flourish with new growth fueled by the parent, extensive roots develop over one or two seasons (depending on the plant type). This allows time for the mother and clone to develop strong shared vascular connections. Then, by carefully cutting at the rooting point, both plants benefit— the mother remains vibrantly nourished, while the generously rooted clone establishes quickly on its own. Through this nurturing natural process, you replenish your medicinal plants generously without compromising the longevity of their valued parent stock. Layering offers herb gardening sustainability through abundant, lush regeneration.

Division of Perennial Herbs

To keep herbaceous perennials thriving for years, dividing plant roots every few seasons refreshes and reinvigorates them. As the central parts grow less vigorous compared to the outer shoots, it's a natural time. Herbs like bee balm, mint, oregano, and lemon balm show this through decreased flowering. In the fall or early spring, before growth starts, dig up the entire root-ball. Remove excess soil and gently separate divisions with clean tools, keeping plenty of roots intact on each piece without tearing. Reset divisions at a similar depth to the parent. After watering thoroughly until they're established, they'll regrow vigorously. Division stimulates new root and shoot regeneration to prevent exhaustion. It's a meditative ritual that reciprocates plants' healing gifts while promoting long-term sustainability in your herb patch.

Special Considerations for Perennial Herbs

When it comes to perennial herbs, propagation requires some different care than annuals. While one-season plants focus solely on blooming and seeding, perennials have a longer life-span and growth pattern to consider. They first concentrate on developing strong root systems before flowering; this takes time compared to quick-germinating annuals. Understanding a perennial's phased progression helps with multiplication. Rather than exhausting themselves with single-season fertility like annuals, sturdy perennials recur year after year. They prioritize establishing deep roots for longevity before repro-ducing above ground. Attending to a perennial's prolonged life cycle results in resilient, long-term colonies through propaga-tion matched to its natural rhythms and needs.

Perennial Growth Habits

Perennial herbs don't always bloom in their first year. In their initial season, their focus is on the underground—building sturdy root foundations. Only in the second year will you start seeing robust leafy top growth and spreading, crowded stems above ground. With strong roots anchoring them by then, plants can store adequate energy through photosynthesis. Most perennials flower reliably in their third season once mature. Some, especially long-lived varieties like echinacea and oregano, may remain productive for over a decade before their vigor naturally declines with age and needs a propagation boost. Understanding an herb's multi-year development cycle from seeds or divisions helps you establish thriving plants able to flower and spread year after year for prolonged harvests.

It takes time for perennial herbs to reach their peak potency and harvest potential through natural growth phases. Consecutive seasons enable deeper root systems to absorb more minerals from soil and store nutrition made in leaves through sun exposure. Flowering then expresses fully ripened chemistry. Propagating via division, layering, or cuttings works best when timed with transitional points in this inherent sequence, like after good rooting or when energy shifts above ground. Understanding variances between species also curbs impatience; some simply take longer to solidify before delivering therapeutic benefits. By mirroring the natural progression tailored to each plant's needs, we support our herbal allies' ease of prolific proliferation over the long haul through propagation in step with their inherent rhythms.

Timing and Seasonal Considerations

Perennial herbs store a lot of energy underground to survive the winter. So, the best times to propagate are late fall through very early spring. As seasons change, plants begin shifting resources from root reserves into flowering or new leafy growth. Their hormones respond to these seasonal cues, jumpstarting regeneration processes. Division, layering, or cuttings can harness this natural productive energy that's already flowing within the herb. Propagating during these windows means taking advantage of the plant's willingness to branch out and establish itself. It's an opportune time when perennials are biologically primed to redirect their strength into multiplying and expanding their colonies for the coming growing season.

As fall arrives, plants get ready for winter by pulling nutrients from leaves back underground. The roots and bases of perennials become well-insulated stores of valuable minerals and energy reserves. By springtime, all that stored-up goodness fuels a burst of new growth from buds just waking up. Young stems can quickly leaf out while root reserves remain high. This makes early spring the perfect season to propagate, whether dividing plant crowns, layering stems, or taking cuttings. By summer, the plant's focus shifts to blooming and seeding instead of recovering from propagation like in the spring. So, timing your efforts for this natural transition gives new clones the head start they need to take root and thrive on their own.

Some herbs that need warmth to flourish, like ginger, turmeric, and arrowroot, can be cloned through their underground storage organs like bulbils, tubers, or rhizome pieces in late summer. While these tropicals are typically perennial, cloning allows treating them as heat-loving annuals anywhere. The key is paying attention to your zone and each plant's natural cues for when to divide; some may be cued by cooling nights, while others respond to dropping day lengths. By syncing propagation methods to an herb's inherent seasonal rhythms, your cloning attempts become a dance perfectly calibrated to the unique characteristics of each medicinal perennial. Letting regional conditions and a plant's internal clock guide you ensures your propagation success and the abundance of healing homegrown remedies.

Caring for Seedlings

Baby herb plants need extra care since they are tender and vulnerable. Between dangers like drying out, drastic temperature changes, soil fungus attacks, and greedy little bugs, there are plenty of potential pitfalls that could strike down your precious new seedlings before they have a chance to reach their full healing potential. With some easy protective measures, you can really boost their odds of survival. A little bit of vigilance goes a long way, from providing steady warmth and moisture to your seed trays to using floating row covers to keep pests away. Taking basic precautions means your immature medicinal plants will be well-defended as they develop their roots.

Transplanting Seedlings

When your plant babies start to grow their second set of real leaves, it's time to give them a little more space. Their roots will be getting really long by now, so gently take them out of the small starter pots and put them in bigger pots with new soil that has more nutrients. Be very gentle when you do this so you don't break the roots. Let them get used to their new home for a couple of weeks before moving them outside. Start by only putting them outside during the daytime when the sun is out, and bring them back in at night. Slowly increase their time outside over a couple of weeks so they get used to the outdoor weather. Make sure to still water them a little, but not as much. Once they look really strong and healthy outside, it should be safe to plant them in the garden as long as the weather is reliably warm—after the last expected frost.

When you move your plants to their new bigger pots, don't go too big, or the soil will stay soggy. The pots should give the roots enough room to spread out but not be too huge. Plant them at the same level as they were in the small pots. Handle them gently as you refill the new pots with soil, packing them down lightly around the stems. Give them some water afterward. While they're getting used to their new homes, protect them from the hot sun or cold winds with mini-greenhouses, upside-down jars, or partial shade for a few weeks. This helps them adjust gradually. You can also plant different batches of the same plants a few weeks apart. That way, you'll have a longer harvest period instead of everything finishing at once. Staggering them over six weeks means a steady supply of food from your garden.

Watering and Fertilizing Seedlings

While sprouts initially depend on water and minerals from internal seed food reserves, once their real leaves come in, that food runs out fast. Now they need nutrients from the soil and water more than ever. If the soil dries out too much, it stresses the baby roots and leaves, which slows how fast they grow and makes them more likely to get sick. But soil that stays too soggy is just as bad—the roots can't breathe if the soil is soaked. Soggy soil also encourages mold and fungus problems. The best soil for them is moist but not soaked, like soft, rich loamy dirt that holds water well without becoming mud. Aim for soil that is damp, not dripping wet or bone dry.

Plants that get a lot of sun will need water more often than ones in shade since the sun helps them make more food through their leaves. Check the soil and leaves every day. If they start to look droopy or yellowish, it's time to water. Do it early in the morning so the plants have all day to dry out before dark. Let a little bit of water drain out of the bottom so you know it's moist enough down below too. Make sure everything dries completely by nighttime to avoid fungus or mildew forming. After about a month of growth in their new locations, you can start giving them diluted liquid fertilizer plant food once a week. Use only half the amount it recommends; that way, you can get them used to the nutrients without burning their young root systems.

Disease and Pest Management

As your plants grow, keep an eye on things like water, air circulation, sunlight, and cleanliness to avoid disease vectors. If any bugs or snails show up, deal with them carefully. Pick off infested leaves and use barriers like copper strips to stop snails. You can also gently spray away small insects. You may avoid slugs and insects by using floating cloth row coverings. Planting some calendulas and dill around the edges attracts helpful predators like wasps that eat other bugs before they can damage plants. Always make sure you know exactly what's bugging your plants before trying anything. Then try the softest methods first, like insecticidal soaps, plant oils, or Bacillus thuringiensis bacteria for wormy caterpillars. Those natural options only target the bad bugs and are safest for the environment.

With attentive observation, prevention, and early intervention, herb seedlings establish gracefully into prolific patches, thriving through seasonal cycles for years on guard duty, promoting your household's holistic health!

<h1 style="text-align:center">Chapter 5</h1>

<h1 style="text-align:center">Essential Medicinal Herbs to Grow</h1>

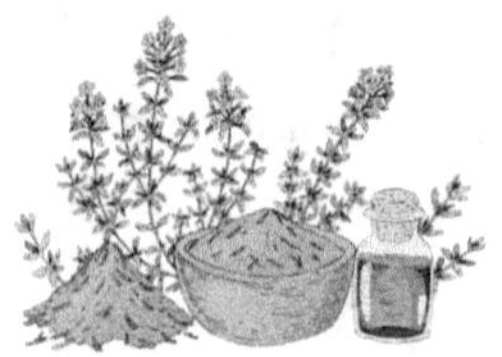

Now that you understand how to prepare fertile growing conditions and propagate resilient herbs successfully, an exciting journey begins—choosing which precious botanical allies to welcome into your wellness sanctuary! With thousands of options spanning the medicinal plant kingdom, deciding the most valuable, versatile, and cherished varieties for your apothecary garden seems like an epic task.

Calendula, lemon balm, sage, thyme, and other treasured herbs provide many medicinal benefits for both beginner and seasoned gardeners. More uncommon forms of motherwort, mullein, astragalus, goldenseal, and potent nightshade family members further expand your herbal medicine repertoire. As you turn through, embrace a few fresh allies; you might notice a bloom that calls out to you to cultivate.

A carefully curated selection of essential medicinal herbs should aim for holistic coverage, balancing sometimes competing approaches to wellness: Calming and stimulating, warming and cooling, drawing poisons, and supporting blood flow. With an attuned gardener's intuitive pull toward helpful plants as your guide, may more abundant health take root!

Profiling Key Herbs and Their Uses

Some really cool medicinal herbs you should think about growing are very helpful for your health and easy to take care of. They're simple to cultivate, so even if you've never gardened before, you'll have fun and success with them. Plus, they look beautiful in your yard or garden. Whether you're a plant rookie or an expert, these herbs will fill you with positive energy and keep your body feeling happy and balanced naturally. Their therapeutic powers are amazing gifts to welcome into your space.

Echinacea—Immune Strengthening Warrior

Echinacea is an awesome Native American healing herb that supports your immune system like nothing else. It contains powerful antioxidants, antiviral, and anticancer ingredients to fight infections, inflammation, and illness. Beyond boosting immunity, it improves lymph flow, speeds wound healing, and builds collagen for healthy skin too. An interesting thing about this herb is that, in its first year, the plant focuses on root growth underground. Then, in the second year, it sends up a basal rosette of leaves. Finally, by the third season, it presents colorful blooms with drooping pink, purple, or white petals circling a copper center. Once established, echinacea spreads easily through self-seeding and easily dividing clumps.

It's easy to grow echinacea, also known as the coneflower, in your backyard. It likes soil that isn't too sandy or clay-like but has some organic material to keep it moist. Most types do well in the sun, like in a spot that gets morning light. You'll have to protect some of the more delicate kinds if you live where it gets cold in the spring, or the flower buds won't form. Echinacea is hardy and can withstand winter in most parts of North America with a layer of mulch. You can start new plants from seeds and root cuttings or divide existing ones. When the flowers are at their peak, cut the whole plant to either tincture fresh for quick relief from colds and flu or dry it to have on hand to boost your immune system during sickness seasons. Echinacea is easy to grow and makes a great natural medicine right in your garden!

Lavender—Fragrant Healer Beloved for Ages

Lavender is another amazing plant to grow in your garden. Not only does it look beautiful with its long-lasting purple flowers in summer, but it also smells incredibly good! The flowers give off a floral scent that can help reduce stress and anxiety. Lavender is really good for you too; it contains powerful oils that can fight infections and ward off bugs. Rubbing lavender oil into your muscles helps relax tension and adding it to baths can soothe your stomach if you're feeling sick. Some people even use lavender to help regulate their menstrual cycle. No wonder herbalists have loved lavender for thousands of years across different cultures.

Lavender grows well when propagated from cuttings. It absolutely loves hot, dry climates similar to areas around the Mediterranean Sea, with cool but not freezing winter temperatures. Lavender does best in soil that drains quickly and is a little alkaline, with a pH level between 6.7 and 7.3. Ensure sharp drainage, avoiding winter moisture sitting on roots that rot plants. For lots of bushy growth, cut the spent flower spikes off after the flowers have finished blooming. You can use the pretty purple flowers, fresh or dried, to make herbal tea, bath products, room sprays, and more. But for the strongest scent, distill the essential oil from the flower spikes. Take time to appreciate lavender with all your senses—its beauty to look at, soothing scent to smell, and relaxation benefits to feel.

Calendula—Sunny Healing Blossoms

Calendula is a cheerful orange flower that loves to spread around gardens. Also called "pot marigold," it blooms non-stop, providing healing benefits. Known as the "poor man's saffron" for its saffron-like color, calendula has anti-inflammatory and antifungal properties. Both the petals and oils help reduce swelling and irritation, both internally and externally. If you get a cut, burn, or rash, just mash up the fresh petals into a paste and apply it as a poultice. You can also infuse them into oil or cream. This makes an excellent natural remedy for wounds. The pretty petals also add color, taste, and preservative qualities if you make herbal skin creams, teas, or syrups yourself.

Calendula is easy to grow because it reseeds easily year after year. Plant the seeds directly in the garden from early spring through mid-summer for continuous blooms. It likes fertile, well-draining soil and full sun. Deadhead any flowers that are wilting to encourage the plant to keep flowering, right up until the first fall frost. The resilient flowers can stay open and closed every day for over a month per plant, as long as you water them regularly and pick them up promptly. At the first sign of an infection, apply a calendula cream or poultice for natural healing. Or keep some in your medicine cabinet for soothing relief whenever inflammation strikes.

Chamomile—Gentle Soother

Chamomile is one of the most well-known calming herbs. Both German and Roman chamomile have been used for centuries to aid digestion, relaxation, and sleep. This ground-covering plant has pretty fern-like leaves and small white daisy flowers. Chamomile contains mild sedative and anti-inflammatory compounds that help soothe upset tummies and irritated skin and reduce stress and anxiety. It's the perfect natural remedy for calming fussy babies or anytime you need relief from an upset stomach or to wind down for sleep. That's why chamomile has been a beloved medicinal herb for so long.

Chamomile grows best in full sun and moderately fertile soil that drains well. Add some lime to adjust the pH to around 6.7–7.2, which chamomile prefers. You can plant the seeds directly where you want them in late spring or early summer because seedlings don't like being moved after sprouting. Chamomile will then spread on its own through self-seeding. Snip the newly opened flowers to enjoy as a delicious, calming tea. You can also extract the essential oils for aromatherapy purposes. For maximum healing benefits, pick the flowers in the morning when they are freshly opened. At this time, they contain higher levels of the oil chamazulene, which is great for fighting allergies and menstrual cramps. Let graceful chamomile flowers decorate your garden and first aid kit with their gentle, soothing properties.

Rosemary—Evergreen Memory Booster

Rosemary is a beautiful evergreen herb that looks great in the garden, on your patio in a pot or braided together for wreaths and decorations. With its pine-scented grayish-green needle-like leaves and light blue flowers, it adds natural beauty wherever you grow it. Roast lamb or chicken with rosemary for amazing flavor. But did you know rosemary is also great for your brain? Sniffing cut sprigs or rosemary vinegar enhances memory and learning, as folk wisdom says. Scientists now know that compounds in rosemary protect brain cells and boost focus (Rahbardar and Hosseinzadeh, 2020). Rosemary's antimicrobial powers also preserve meat and prevent wine from oxidizing quickly. That's why Greeks wore rosemary wreaths while studying for mental sharpness—it really works! Whether cooking or studying, let versatile rosemary enhance both body and mind.

Rosemary does best in very well-draining soil, so plant it on sloping ground or in raised beds. It can even grow in poorer soil. Make sure the pH is around 6.7 and it gets full sun. Protect rosemary from harsh winter cold snaps. In hot summers, occasionally water it deeply, as rosemary doesn't like wet feet. Prune it once a year to keep it bushy and encourage new growth. Propagate rosemary from stem cuttings in early summer. Harvest the leaves right before the flowers open for cooking and wellness purposes. With its brain-boosting powers and tasty additions to food, resinous rosemary is worth growing to nourish both mind and body.

Lemon Balm—Uplifting Restorative

Lemon balm is known as a plant friend that soothes both the body and mind. If someone you care about isn't feeling well, lemon balm can help in many gentle ways. Its aromatic leaves contain compounds that relieve anxiety, calm upset tummies, and fight cold sores with antiviral power. Steeping the bright green wrinkly leaves as tea or tincture chills you out, reduces fevers, and promotes relaxing sleep—you'll feel its calming effects. Even just inhaling lemon balm's sunny citrus scent noticeably lifts your mood. As one of the easiest herbs to grow, its shallow roots divide easily so you'll have plenty.

Lemon balm thrives with reliable watering in everyday garden soil, in partial or full sun. It sprouts quickly from seeds or root cuttings and will spread around happily if the conditions are good. To manage the plant and keep it from taking over, pick the leaves often for various uses. Chop fresh lemon balm to brighten fruit salads, herbal teas, honey, and homemade drinks. When creating herbal remedies, the leaves are most potent right before flowering, when the aromatic oils are concentrated —perfect for infused oil extracts. Rely on cheerful lemon balm to lift your mood and calm anxieties all summer.

Sage—Cleansing and Clearing

Sage has beautiful grayish-green leaves and vivid spring flowers that buzzing bees love. This hardy plant returns year after year, providing more than just tasty flavor when cooking chicken or turkey. According to folklore, sage also offers protective qualities. Scientifically, sage contains powerful anti-inflammatory and antimicrobial compounds that can help balance gut bacteria, clear congestion, calm diarrhea, and fight infection throughout the body (Hamidpour et al., 2014). Its scientific name "Salvia" stems from the Latin word meaning "heal and save," and that's just what it can do. Whether munching on roasted sage or using it medicinally, let sturdy sage enrich your well-being in many soothing ways.

Sage grows quickly from seeds or stem cuttings planted in the spring in well-draining, nutrient-rich soil with lots of sun. It sprouts best when daytime temperatures are around 60–70°F. In very cold climates, sage may need protection over winter to stay thriving for years. Snip the leaves before the plant flowers, when their aromatic oils are at their highest. Of course, sage adds savory flavor to meals, but try refreshing sage baths too, or burning sage for traditional cleansing rituals. You can even use it to help with night sweats. With all its uses for wellness, it's no wonder sage has long been a staple medicinal herb.

Specific Care for Each Herb

Beyond environmental factors like sunlight and drainage matching plant temperaments, individual herbs express preferences for soil nutrition, hydration, pruning times, and harvest techniques based on regional origins and growth habits. Fine-tuning care to align with beloved botanicals' ideal conditions rewards the attentive gardener with vigorous abundance.

Soil and Sun Requirements

Most herbs grow well in average fertile loam soils with sand-to-clay loam textures with slight acidity and a neutral pH of around 6.5. But some prefer certain conditions that match where they naturally live. Herbs from grasslands like echinacea and rosemary want soil amended with limestone to raise the pH closer to 7. Herbs growing in forests, such as goldenseal, bloodroot, and black cohosh, need acidic leaf compost below 6, like in their native habitat. Thyme and lavender from alkaline lands also appreciate limestone. Don't mix fussy herbs that demand different soil; give them their happy place in the garden instead, like a raised bed.

While some herbs love lots of sun, it's good to see what each one prefers through observation. Some herbs may seem too hot in the full midday sun and do better with morning warmth and afternoon shade. Pay attention to whether the plants seem happy or tired. Their natural habitats can clue you in too; parsley and cilantro want cooler seasons, and basil requires more heat. By giving herbs a sunlight schedule that matches when they naturally do most growing, like more morning sun versus afternoon, you'll prevent them from wilting in too much sun or going into shock from not enough. Experiment to match each herb's sunning habits so they have their perfect conditions without stress.

Watering and Feeding Guidelines

Herbs from dry places like rosemary and thyme dislike wet feet but need deep watering during heat waves. They prefer soil that drains quickly to avoid sogginess. Mixing in sand or gravel around these herbs ensures fast-drying soil. On the other hand, lemon balm, elderberry, and passionflower that grow near streams want regular moisture or they'll droop. Pay attention to where herbs are originally from—desert or riverside. Then mimic their natural watering patterns so roots stay content. Those from arid zones do best with occasional deep soakings in very well-draining soil. Stream herbs appreciate consistent moisture.

Feeding guidelines are also tailored to each herb's hunger. Heavy-feeding annuals like basil, borage, and calendula, have bigger appetites than others. These fast-growing herbs that complete their life cycle in one year do best with nutrient-rich soil boosted regularly with compost. You can also give them a light organic fertilizer each month once they are planted. On the other hand, hardier perennials like oregano, lavender, and sage that return year after year don't want overly rich soil. Too many nutrients can cause these woody herbs to hold too much moisture or flower less. Instead, they thrive in lean, alkaline conditions. See how each herb responds: Vigorous growth means they want food, while lethargy may signal too many nutrients.

Pruning and Harvesting Techniques

Taking good care of your perennial herbs is important to get the most healthy, flavorful harvests. Pruning them back regularly results in thicker, bushier growth that bugs don't like as much. Cut off the older stems near the base so the new shoots get more sun and airflow; this makes the plant stronger. Do your trimming right before flowering when the leaves and buds are at their most potent. Then you can dry the cuttings to enjoy later! Steep them in hot water to make tea, soak them in alcohol to make tinctures, or hang them in a dark, airy place to dry completely. Doing it this way locks in all the aromatic oils and nutrients.

It's important to harvest your herbs the right way at the perfect time to get the most medicine out of them. For example, mint leaves have the most menthol in the morning after the dew dries. In the hot afternoon, plants pull nutrients back down to their roots. Some leaves, like borage and comfrey, are kind of hairy, so remove the thick middle vein before using them. Get to know each plant from when it starts as a seed until it finishes its cycle. Pay attention to how and when different herbs naturally grow. Then you can care for them in a way that matches their true selves and the season. In return, they'll share their healing powers through beauty and what you make from them.

Seasonal Considerations

Attending the medicinal garden through seasonal transitions allows herbs to shine fully from seed to harvest. Spring preparation welcomes new growth; summer nurturing rewards a bounty for preserving into winter rest. Each phase demands certain care when herbs commune most vibrantly with us.

Spring Preparation and Planting

When winter finally lets go, you start getting excited for the colorful growing season ahead! This is the time when gardening heats up. You get your garden beds ready by pulling any weeds and fluffing up the soil so it's nice and fertile. It's also smart to start your seeds indoors, where it's warmer until the chance of frost passes. Putting up stakes, mulch, and trellises beforehand helps prevent future clutter and confusion. The mulch locks moisture in the ground, and stakes and trellises give vines and tall plants something to climb up, so everything has room to spread out nicely within its space. With a little prep work now, your plants will be happy and healthy all season!

Certain herbs like cool weather best, so plant them first as the soil slowly gets warmer. Hardy annuals that reseed themselves, like cilantro, borage, calendula, and dill, can go directly into the ground after the last frost when it's reliably over 50 degrees Fahrenheit. You'll also transplant any seedlings you started indoors earlier, but ease them outside slowly over a week so they can adjust to the sun. Think about how tall each herb will get and space them out accordingly so they don't get over-crowded as they grow. It's also key to pull any weeds right away so they don't steal nutrients and space from your herb seedlings as their roots take hold.

Summer Growth and Maintenance

Now that the warmer weather has everything growing like crazy, your garden is bursting with life and promise! This busy period means keeping up with watering, pruning to shape plants and boost productivity, and keeping an eye out for any bugs or weeds sneaking in. Some taller herbs, like angelica, and some echinacea varieties might need stakes so big storms don't knock them over. Also, make sure your flowering plants have plenty of space so nothing feels crowded. As the sun moves across the sky each day, rotate potted herbs to the brightest spots. A bit of tending goes a long way to keep things looking neat and prevent problems, even when nature's in full hype mode.

In the height of summer, focus on picking flavorful leaves and flowers from herbs like anise hyssop, calendula, borage, lemon balm, and holy basil before they start focusing energy on making seeds. Cutting them earlier sometimes gets you more blooms too. But if flowers have just opened, it's better to leave them to fully ripen into seeds. Pay attention to each plant's unique stage to know the best time—are the leaves or flowers at their peak? Knowing an herb's natural rhythms helps you harvest it at its peak for maximum flavor, beauty, and health benefits. Summer offers such an amazing variety of gifts from your garden if you respect each plant's authentic schedule.

Fall Harvest and Winter Care

As summer waves say goodbye with one last colorful display, fall arrives, offering a bounty before everything goes dormant for winter. Now is the perfect time to collect roots, berries, and some seeds from herbs like dandelion, echinacea, marshmallow, and chaste tree; their medicine is at peak potency just before hibernating. Clean up dead foliage to add to your compost pile, leaving behind reminders of each plant's full cycle. Give tender perennials or seedlings you want to overwinter extra protection under a cold frame. Mulch around hardy plants like rosemary, thyme, and sage to minimize freezing. Take a moment to feel proud of all you grew and gathered through careful tending across the changing seasons. Then, relax as your garden rests, learning from the past year while envisioning next spring's possibilities!

Sustainable Harvesting Practices

It's smart of an herbalist to remember that everything is connected. So, when picking plants, think about helping both them and the environment stay balanced. Harvest wild herbs in a way that keeps populations healthy, like only taking some from diverse areas. And grow your own using methods that support the plants, like rotating the parts you collect so they can fully regrow. This symbiotic approach keeps your healing greens coming back stronger each season while supporting all the wildlife and ecosystems they're part of too. Their gifts keep flowing when we care for the whole network in a mindful way.

Understanding Sustainable Harvesting

When gathering herbs from nature, it's important to form a respectful relationship that benefits both people and plants. Consider each herb's habitat requirements and ability to reproduce fully each season so the supply stays plentiful. Different areas may have more or less herbs, depending on yearly weather patterns. Select common, resilient plants at their peak to take only what you need without depleting future growth. Gather selectively from patches that look thriving, versus emptying smaller groups. This ensures the land and its herbal inhabitants remain balanced and fruitful for generations. Forming thoughtful partnerships with plants allows enjoying nature's pharmacy sustainably for both people and the earth.

When foraging herbs, only collect a little from each thriving patch—around 10% or less. Take whole plants sparingly, leaving most to continue growing. Let some seed heads fully mature for birds and small animals to eat, scattering the rest in suitable areas to spread new herbs. Visit different harvesting spots each year instead of emptying the same places repeatedly.

In between visits, remove any invasive weeds that could damage diversity over time. By giving back through gentle nurturing of herb habitats between visits, nature's healing botanical bounty can enrich us sustainably over the long term.

By simply planting even a small herb garden at home, you can grow many of the plants you might otherwise collect from the wild. This reduces pressure on delicate ecosystems and native habitats. And when you do spend time in nature, focus on connecting with healing plants spiritually rather than just gathering piles. Nurturing rare plants at home, like ginseng, also safeguards them from being stolen or over-harvested. Overall, having an outdoor green space to sustainably cultivate useful herbs meets your wellness needs harmoniously. It reduces reliance on wild-picking while deepening your understanding and respect for these gifts of nature. With mindful growing and collecting, we cherish the earth's herbs respectfully for generations to come.

Planting for Continual Harvest

For an ongoing supply of fresh herbs throughout the summer, plant favorites like dill, cilantro, parsley, and basil in batches every four weeks so they're ready to pick, one after the other. Perennial herbs like sage, thyme, and oregano get tired after flowering, so shear them back to encourage more leaf growth later in the fall. Plant garlic, onions, and fennel bulbs close together too since they will multiply below the soil each season, giving a bigger harvest. With a little successive sowing and pruning of herbs, you can enjoy fresh flavor and medicine for much longer instead of everything bolting at once.

It's smart to rotate which herbs grow in each garden bed from year to year. Dedicate areas to plant families like alliums, mustards, or nightshades. This avoids exhausting the soil nutrients any one group needs or passing on potential pests and bugs. You can also plant green manure crops or let bee-friendly weeds grow between harvesting seasons. Things like alfalfa, clover, and dandelions enrich the earth naturally. Then the next herbs you sow will thrive with extra nutrients and minerals. Taking turns using the soil and letting it replenish keeps it vibrant long-term.

Taking care of the land is important. Weeding out invasive species that crowd out native plants helps preserve habitats. Partnering with local conservation groups is cool too; we can learn from them while contributing to their important work. Being an herbalist is about more than just using plants ourselves. It's recognizing that human health depends on the health of the ecosystems and communities around us.

Chapter 6

Garden Maintenance and Troubleshooting

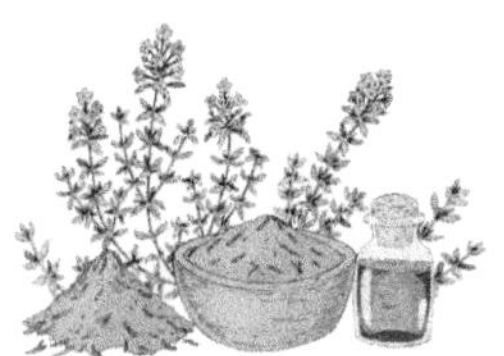

Even the most conscientious gardeners encounter challenges with weather, pests, or simple oversights that can quickly escalate if left unchecked. Maintaining vigilant observation paired with prompt supportive care gently realigns balance. Troubleshooting common herb garden issues as learning opportunities deepens adaptive stewardship practice through each season.

Exploring diverse integrated approaches will hopefully spark creative strategies and empathy for all beings. The herbalist aims for prevention first, careful monitoring next, and minimally disruptive amendments as indicated. Sometimes losses occur—an early freeze, a careless lawn mower, or a hungry deer. We mourn and then learn from every experience. Maybe keep a garden notebook where you can jot down observations, remedies attempted, and resolutions.

Stewarding a garden brings us face-to-face with nature's authentic, imperfect essence—much less pristine than photos often portray. Yet within reality's vibrant complexity lies deeper insights if we look beneath surface views. Why is that wilted? Who benefits from this challenge? The back-and-forth interchanges within ecosystems and between us and the living landscapes to which we tend offer life's greatest tutelage if we open our awareness. Challenges arise not to discourage but to deepen our relationships and understanding and strengthen diverse members of the community over the long run. May this planting guide help you and your treasured green companions care for one another with knowledge and care through the seasons.

Watering and Nutrient Management

Taking good care of your herbal plants requires paying close attention to their watering and nutrition needs. Each herb has different requirements to stay happy and healthy. When herbs thrive, their leaves, flowers, and other parts contain the strongest levels of beneficial compounds. This allows them to offer the best possible medicine. To do that, we need to understand what watering and feeding each plant prefers. By providing just the right amounts, you help herbs reach their full potential.

Proper Watering Techniques

To properly water your herbs, you need to understand each plant's individual needs as well as how different conditions affect soil moisture levels. Things like weather, soil properties, and the plant's current development stage influence how much and how often they need water. Rather than sticking to a set schedule, adjust your approach according to the situation. Pay attention to signs of dryness in the herbs themselves and in the soil. Frequent, shallow watering may suit some plants, while others prefer deeper water less often. Tailoring your technique this way means meeting each herb's requirements for ideal hydration and growth at every stage, from seedling to harvest.

Watering Frequency and Depth

When it comes to watering most herbs, consistency is key. They tend to do best with regular moisture in the soil rather than swings between extremes of too wet or dry. Aim to water when the top few inches start drying out, but before it gets completely parched. As a baseline, watering two to three times per week when rain is lacking works well. But adjust according to your conditions; soil type and climate make a difference. Loamy soil may dry out faster, warranting daily sprinkles versus heavier, fewer waterings for clay. Similarly, herbs in hot spots need more frequent drinks. Observe how quickly moisture leaves each area. Tailoring your routine ensures herbs stay content without stress from underwatering or sogginess.

For optimal watering, make sure you thoroughly soak the whole root area of each herb plant. Aim to moisten the soil down to at least six inches deep whenever you water. Slow, deep watering is preferable to frequent light sprinkles. The reason is that wetting the entire root zone encourages roots to grow downward, searching for moisture reserves. This results in herbs with stronger, healthier root structures. Plants with deep roots can better withstand hot, dry stretches since they can tap into subterranean water supplies.

Adjusting Watering Based on Plant Needs and Weather Conditions

Not all herbs have the same thirst. Various factors impact individual water needs, so it's smart to observe closely. Some, like rosemary and oregano, naturally tolerate dry spells better than others that crave constant moisture, like mints. Climate and weather also affect soil hydration. Mediterranean herbs planted in your regions may need less than expected. And a string of rainy days means less watering than usual hot stretches. Rather than follow a set schedule, check in on plants and soil regularly.

On extra-hot days, herbs need more water to make up for what the sun pulls out rapidly through transpiration. When temperatures soar, give your plants an extra drink to prevent wilting and stress. Also, aim to water in the evening rather than in the blazing heat of the afternoon. This gives herbs all night long to absorb moisture before another scorcher arrives. Conversely, cut back on watering when it's mainly cool, overcast, or rainy for a stretch. Less sun means less moisture loss, so too much water could saturate their soil. Adjust your habits to suit diverse conditions.

Nutrient Requirements

In addition to proper watering, medicinal herb plants need adequate nutrition from the soil to produce robust growth and high concentrations of active medicinal compounds. Organic fertilizers and amendments tailored to an individual herb's needs are ideal for providing long-term soil nutrition without synthetics.

Understanding Specific Nutrient Needs

Herbs vary in their tastes when it comes to nutrients, just like their water preferences. Those evolved to flourish in scarce conditions, such as thyme from rocky hillsides, thrive on minimal nutrition. Too much food, in contrast, can dilute the strong qualities we grow them for by promoting fast, weak development at the cost of concentration. Meanwhile, powerhouses like mint that demand generous feeding come alive with supplements like compost or natural fertilizer applied sparingly at first. Pay attention to an herb's evolutionary background to determine how rich its desires are.

Doing your research pays off big time when preparing soil for medicinal herbs. Find out what key nutrients each variety thrives on best, so you know what to aim for. Then choose fertilizers and amendments tailored perfectly to meet specific needs. For example, calcium and magnesium make bee balm sing, so mixing dolomitic lime into its particular soil ensures superb flowering and medicinal content. Rather than generic tosses of this and that, target each plant's blueprint for strength by focusing amendments on what fuels its inner machinery.

Implementing Organic Fertilizers and Soil Amendments

The secrets to growing thriving herbs are in the soil. Create nutrient-rich earth by amending your garden beds with organic matter like aged manure, compost, and green manure crops. Well-decomposed manure supplies a balanced trio of nitrogen, phosphorus, and potassium nutrients over time. Compost adds beneficial microbes along with essential minerals. Letting clover or buckwheat grow and then tilling it into the soil feeds the underground ecosystem. You can also use targeted natural amendments like rock phosphate or greensand to provide specific nutrients as needed by different plants.

With a little effort each year, you can transform your soil into a nourishing environment for medicinal herbs. Aim to work two to four inches of compost or other organic matter into garden beds annually. This improves the texture and nutrient content of the earth over time. By getting the soil right, your plants will thrive. Be attentive with watering methods too to keep roots happy. Mastering soil nutrition through organic amendments tailored to each herb's needs allows you to unlock their full therapeutic power.

Mulching and Weed Control

Properly mulching and managing weeds are essential skills for any medicinal herb gardener. The use of mulch conserves soil moisture, moderates soil temperatures, and inhibits weed growth. Pairing mulch with manual weed removal and weed-blocking ground covers offers an integrated, natural approach to keeping medicinal herb beds weed-free and thriving.

Mulching Strategies

Using organic mulch around your medicinal herbs has many advantages. Mulch helps the soil retain moisture, so the herbs need watering less frequently. It insulates shallow roots from extreme heat or cold by moderating temperature swings in the earth. As the mulch material, like wood chips or grass clippings, breaks down over time, it enriches the soil by improving its texture and providing extra nutrients. The mulch layer protects herbs while also requiring less effort on your part. With this simple addition, moisture levels stay optimal, and your plants get the consistent growing conditions they need to thrive without fussing over water and temperature fluctuations.

Naked dirt loses water quickly when exposed to sun and wind —the evaporation rate can be up to five times higher without coverage. But mulch changes that. A two-to-four-inch layer shields the ground from the sun and wind, slowing evaporation. Instead of surface drying, rainfall, and watering infiltrate deeper. This gives herb roots more time to take up water and nutrients, even in drier spells. With a mulch barrier, the soil stays moist longer, so you can cut back on watering. This extra organic material sparks microbe activity too, which creates healthier soil. As mulch decomposes, it enhances drainage and air pockets while also boosting the earth's ability to hold nutrients. Continuous mulching progressively builds more robust, fertile dirt, perfectly suited for medicinal herbs. Instead of being a single-season solution, mulch nourishes the ground long-term as an integral part of the ecosystem.

When picking a mulch, steer clear of anything dyed or made from chemically processed wood; you want something natural that improves the soil rather than potentially harming it. Look for mulches that will safely break down over time, suppress weeds, and feed the earth. Excellent organic choices are well-rotted compost, shredded hardwood bark, wood chips, fallen leaves, straw, or grass clippings free of seeds. Focus on eco-friendly materials that allow herbs to thrive without risks from harmful additives or pollutants.

Both compost and shredded bark make excellent mulches, but each has advantages. Compost feeds the soil well as it gently breaks down, while bark hangs on longer. Compost holds water terrifically but replenishes the earth a bit faster than bark. Bark provides steady nutrients as it disintegrates sluggishly. Both styles keep herb beds looking tidy. Or go for a shaggier look with wood chips, leaves, or straw; they allow for a more natural scene. Test diverse materials, seeing how each affects moisture holding, weeds, and plant growth in your particular gardens. With a little trial and error, you'll discover the ideal mulch match for optimizing your herbs' health wherever they grow.

Weed Prevention and Management

Mulch goes a long way, but some weeds will still find their way into herb beds. To stay on top of them, regular hand weeding is key. Small, young weeds are easiest—pull them before their roots run deep. It's worth getting proper tools to help with the job too. Keep trowels and knife-like weeders handy for digging around roots and levering them free from soil. A hand fork also pries out pesky invaders. Spending a little time de-weeding periodically, especially after it rains, can prevent patches from forming. With the right removal technique and tools, mulch plus careful attention lets you and your herbs stay on top of unwanted plants.

To stay on top of weeds, start pulling regularly before any have a chance to go to seed. Soil is easiest to work on after rain when roots slip out without breaking. Handle weeds gently to minimize soil disruption and root pieces getting left behind. Even tiny fragments can reproduce problem plants like dandelions. If you can, extract all of the root system when weeding, or else you'll be at it constantly as regrowth occurs. Develop weeding into a routine habit for clean, healthy herb beds without persistent invaders.

When pulling weeds that haven't fully flowered yet, seal them in bags rather than putting immature seeds into compost. Those weeds could sprout up later from compost spread in gardens. It's also smart to define clear edges for planted spaces versus paths or lawns. Try maintaining herb beds within contained ringed plots and containers, or use landscape fabric under plantings. Sharp edges make it much easier to spot and pull only the weeds invading garden areas. Separating zones simplifies the whole weeding process.

Beyond vigilant mulching and weeding, certain living ground covers can further inhibit weed encroachment by outcompeting invaders. Effective options include native violets, wild strawberries, thyme, creeping raspberries, sedums, and miniature clovers like Dutch white. These tough, spreading plants choke out space and starve emerging weed seedlings.

Some herb varieties, like mint, will function as living mulches. Within their preferred growing conditions, vigorous mint quickly fills space, crowding weeds. Plant other herbs within the mint beds to benefit from the weed-suppressing capabilities of these aggressive plants. Opt for mint companions that won't mind moist, fertile soil and partial shade from expansive mint canopies.

Combining organic mulch with manual weeding and weed-blocking ground covers offers the best containment strategy. A multi-tactic defense keeps invasive plants from stealing water, nutrients, and light from vulnerable medicinal herbs. With consistent monitoring and environmentally sustainable practices, herb gardeners can help valuable medicinal plants claim their rightful space to fully thrive.

Pest and Disease Management

Growing healthy medicinal herbs relies heavily on effective organic prevention and management of pests and diseases. Careful monitoring for early signs of trouble allows for targeted treatment to support plant vitality without harmful chemicals.

Identifying Common Garden Pests

It pays to keep a watchful eye on medicinal herbs for any pest problems before they get out of hand. The sooner you spot issues like nibbled leaves or bug clusters, the better the chance of effective control with minimal impact on plants. Don't wait until damage is widespread to take action. Understanding helpful predators in the garden also helps natural methods work better. You can encourage good bugs to eat damaging ones.

Recognizing Signs of Pest Damage

Chewing insects will leave holes with ragged edges in the leaves. Small sucking bugs cause mottled or wilted leaves, yellowing, and plants not reaching their full size. Always look beneath the foliage too, as tiny pests hide there. Larvae and critters lurk on the undersides, where they're harder to notice. Caterpillars can defoliate plants shockingly fast. Overnight, they might strip plants bare if not addressed right away.

Some pests wreak havoc below the soil. Collapsing or weak plants could mean maggots munching roots. Watch out too for ant trails near plant bases; those often signal scale bugs or aphids that ants protect. Even subtle signs deserve a closer look. If herbs seem generally unwell without cause, that warrants doing some sleuthing at the root level for potential culprits.

Beneficial Insects for Natural Pest Control

Rather than harsh chemicals, recruit helpful predators to eat damaging bugs for you! Ladybugs, green lacewings, and tiny Trichogramma wasps are good bugs who gobble up common garden threats. By planting tasty blooms like sweet alyssum, cosmos, and parsley, they'll stick around to protect your plants. Diverse flowers offer shelter and food to keep these natural defenders thriving. Plus, they'll keep working all season without cost.

Strategically placed birdhouses, bat boxes, bird baths, and overwintering sites also encourage pest-eating wildlife to take up residence in the garden. Nature provides these built-in checks and balances when space is made for helpful allies.

Organic Approaches to Pest Management

Where pest populations overwhelm nature's defenses, organic treatments can reduce their numbers without toxic chemicals. Methods like companion planting, physical barriers, traps, and homemade sprays target problematic insects and small animals effectively.

Companion Planting for Pest Prevention

You can outsmart pests just by clever plant pairing. Some herbs have nature's bug repellent built right in. Strong scents from onions, chives, garlic, or marigolds disguise plants from chomp-happy insects. You can also plant decoys to be dinner instead of your priority produce. Nasturtiums or dill happily entertain diners, sparing other herbs from being gobbled up. Let the trap crops play snack patrol. Meanwhile, their tempting scents keep bug appetites away from key culinary or medicinal plants.

Want nature's best cops on pest patrol? Tuck flowers throughout your herb beds. This invites in ladybugs, lacewing bugs, tiny wasps, and fly allies that snack all season on annoying aphids and caterpillars. Shelter these good guys among herbs they can zip between on bug-busting sprees. Help them thrive by avoiding sprays that harm all bugs alike. Also give predators places to hide out of harm's way, like under leaf litter or between plant stems.

Homemade Remedies for Pest Control

If companion planting isn't enough and pests gain ground, there are softer solutions. Try insecticidal soaps, neem oil, or plant oils to tame troublemakers without harming good bugs. These natural sprays break down fast, so you don't poison your bug allies. For stubborn omnivores like caterpillars or beetles, look for selective bacteria products containing Bacillus thuringiensis (Bt). Only chewing eaters are susceptible, so you won't disrupt pollinators or predator populations like you would with harsh chemicals.

Traps catch pests before they multiply. Colorful sticky boards lure winged invaders to give you a bug body count, so you know just what problems need addressing. Plant collars, netting, or row covers also block common crop munchers. Though prevention is better than cure, traps provide backup by capturing invaders whose physical barriers are missed. Use defense in layers for sustainable protection.

Recognizing and Addressing Common Diseases

Being able to tell diseases apart starts with knowing the signs. Major wilting, or if healthy plants just seem off, could point to problems below ground. Leaf marks, spots, or discoloration usually mean fungi or bacteria are invading the topside. Learning markings unique to diseases lets you pin down the culprit faster. It also helps that moisture-loving pathogens usually strike when there's a wet, warm stretch. After rainfall or high humidity, watch carefully for spreading spots.

Powdery mildew leaves behind a telltale white, powder-like coating when humidity hangs around. Rust diseases erupt as reddish, blister-like spots that rupture from the underside up. Wilting can cause plant roots or circulatory systems to struggle —leaves flop and stems go soft. But causes vary, so diagnosis differs too. Accurately identifying each problem is important to picking the right natural remedies for healing. A milky white coating means sulfur treatments may help a plant fight back. But rust calls for removing blighted foliage or using a plant tonic instead. Proper care starts with the correct naming of what ails each plant.

To avoid the buildup of troublesome pests and diseases, shift around annual herbs in your beds from year to year. For perennials you grow repeatedly, like mint, thyme, and oregano, pick sturdier varieties equipped to resist common afflictions. Flavorful large-leaf basils withstand fusarium and verticillium wilts better than others. Golden marjoram lives on despite root knots and fungus. Hill hardy French tarragon braves root rot in dense soils. Greek columnar oregano stays strong and beautiful during muggy conditions that plague leaf diseases. Always choose robust cultivars that evolved to power through hardships. Duplicate the cleanest, healthiest specimens primed to pass sturdiness down, skipping weaker stock unlikely to weather challenges.

Caught early, proactive prevention and gentle treatment readily resolve many pest and disease issues while safeguarding medicinal herb potency. Establishing a balanced ecosystem empowers nature's defenders to remedy small invasions. With season-long vigilance, resilient plant choices, and sustainable care, you can bolster plant defenses for low-impact harvests of healthy herbs.

Seasonal Maintenance Routines

Growing a flourishing medicinal herb garden relies on consistent, seasonally appropriate care throughout the year. Dedicating time to garden upkeep during each season supports plant health, curtails issues before they spread, and ensures bountiful harvests.

Spring Garden Preparation

Spring is an important season for setting up success before the hectic growing months arrive. Pre-season preparation establishes optimal conditions for vigorous summer herb growth. Begin spring renewal by clearing away old herb stalks, leaves, and mulch from the previous season. These potential hiding spots harbor overwintering pests and disease spores that could reinfect fresh growth if left intact. Safely remove to municipal green waste recycling or burn if permitted.

Once the garden canvas emerges, top the beds with 1-2 inches of finished compost, working it gently into the top few inches of soil to avoid disturbing delicate shallow roots. Compost feeds essential soil microbes and provides a slow-release nutrient source to fuel spring plant growth.

Spring cleaning is the perfect time to stop any troublesome pests or diseases from the get-go as the new season starts. Inspect your herb plants thoroughly as you tidy up. Check crowns and roots for signs of trouble like fungal rot, tiny mites, or other invaders. Nip potential problems in the bud by pruning and tossing any damaged sections or whole plants as needed. Use this fresh start moment to get ahead of ongoing afflictions so your herbs stay in top form to grow and provide medicine or flavoring all summer.

Nip pest issues in the bud early in the season by taking strategic precautions. Slow-moving slugs and snails can be safely removed by hand under moonlight or else trapped before they multiply. Ever-hungry aphids can be deterred using light oil applied while trees rest. Vulnerable plants stay shielded from hungry mouths until they fall out. With a little fore-thought, you can outsmart critters before their minor nibbles turn major. Rather than reacting to crises down the line, low-effort precautions now shield harvests later on.

Summer Growth Monitoring

During the active growing season, regularly walk through and visually assess plants to catch problems early when they are small. Swift preventative care improves outcomes substantially compared to allowing issues to become severe before addressing them. Taking a moment each time to really look at the leaves as you care for your herbs pays off tremendously. Are leaves crinkled from thirst or speckled with issues? Do colors imply too much or too little of certain soil goods? Notice struggling plants or odd symptoms hinting at deeper issues. Tag spots that don't seem right and think detective—what could be the real cause? Over time, keeping notes reveals repeating themes begging for remedies. This approach beats clueless watering and hoping for the best.

Monitor developing flower buds and fruit for disguised guests like tomato hornworms, earwigs, or birds. Install protective netting over ripening seeds and medicinal flowers if needed. Traps help quantify pest pressure to determine effective countermeasures.

Use check-ins to tweak irrigation run times and schedules based on weather fluctuations and plant moisture needs. Deep water established perennial herbs 1-2 times per week in the absence of rain. Increase the frequency of potted plants or seedlings. Apply balanced liquid fertilizer monthly to heavier-feeding plants, transitioning to water only as fall approaches. Address individual plant requirements as observed instead of a fixed regimen.

Practical Troubleshooting

Even seasoned herb gardeners encounter perplexing plant problems. Getting to the root cause of issues can be frustrating, but methodically ruling out variables offers clues. This section covers diagnosing common garden afflictions and delivers targeted troubleshooting advice for nurturing vital medicinal herbs.

Common Garden Issues and Solutions

Interpreting generic symptoms pointing to underlying issues is the first step toward resolutions. Whether dealing with stunted seedlings or sudden plant decline, tracing visible clues back to the source is key for successful interventions.

Plants exhibit general distress in common ways that hint at broader categories to investigate, like water stress, nutrient problems, environmental factors, pests, or disease. Track down the triggers within each realm prompting observable plant reactions.

- **Yellowing leaves:** Investigate soil pH extremes, poor drainage, damaged roots, nutrient deficiencies, pest issues, or natural fall dieback as potential reasons. Identify if problems are isolated or widespread.
- **Wilting foliage:** Rule out underwatering, drought stress, root disruption, transplant shock, pruned roots, or vascular diseases impeding water movement within the plant. Determine if wilting persists at night.
- **Leggy, weak growth:** Suspect insufficient sunlight, overcrowding, excess nitrogen fertilization, wind or cold damage, or root restrictions as possible influences on vigor.

After generally diagnosing problems, consider the unique needs of the affected herbs for tailored solutions. For instance, lavender likes drier soil, yet potted rosemary may require more water than its Mediterranean equivalents. When troubleshooting, take into consideration factors such as growth habits, natural environments, and maturation pace.

- **Basil:** Yellow leaves with green veins typically indicate magnesium deficiencies in fast-growing basils. Apply Epsom salts per label directions to restore color and vigor.
- **Oregano:** Shriveled leaf tips and small leaf size often derive from underwatering. Oregano flourishes with consistent moisture and hot conditions. Ramp up the watering frequency for the best growth.
- **Echinacea:** Powdery white leaf spots signify Echinacea's fungal nemesis, powdery mildew. Improve air circulation and remove infected material to protect healthy tissue. Apply neem oil to deter spread.
- **Lavender:** Silvery foliar discoloration and dieback points to lavender's number one killer: Root rot and fungal issues in heavy, wet soils. Improve drainage or transplant to raised beds to help lavender thrive.

General clues only go so far; really knowing your herbs is key. Tune solutions tightly to each kind's preferred patterns, quirks, and limits uniquely shaped by long ancestry. Familiarize yourself with what's normal and ideal for the varieties in your care. Recognize oddballs from their usual selves. Issues that repeatedly resurface may also stem from situations that do not perfectly match needs. These plants evolved finely tuned to live distinct lives, so honor individuality when troubleshooting.

Preventing Future Problems

An ounce of prevention saves pounds of lost harvests for frustrated herb gardeners. Steer clear of common pitfalls from the start by:

- selecting disease-resistant varieties better adapted to local climate rigors
- providing adequate sunlight and room for each herb to reach mature dimensions
- testing soil and adjusting composition to align with an herb's favored pH and nutrients
- using drip irrigation and mulch for efficient moisture consistency
- monitoring regularly for early signs of stress or encroaching issues

With attentive growing conditions and protective measures built into garden care routines, many difficult herb vexations simply never take root. An observant, proactive systems approach maintains equilibrium for nature to reward the diligent grower with vigorous yields.

Chapter 7

Harvesting Your Herbs

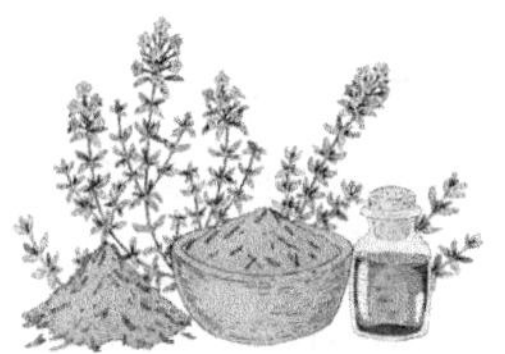

After months of nurturing, the anticipation of harvest arrives! After patiently shepherding delicate baby plants into powerful remedies in greenery form, the moment arrives to gather the rewards. You poured your care into these special beauties as valiant nature concentrated curative forces within bursting blooms and fruits. It's their magical peak, so collect with care and celebrate all your partnership has achieved. Through your green thumb and nature's green magic, health, and vitality, you've grown for yourself and your community. The therapeutic treasures you've partnered to cultivate shall remedy and nourish.

When harvest arrives, your partnership with these healing plants comes full circle. From tiny seeds bursting with promise to flourishing remedies bearing nature's coded treasures, you've faithfully tended their journey according to innate cycles.

While seasonal shifts offer ballpark cues, the best harvest timing calls for devoted observation of personal plant traits. General guidelines only get you so far; knowing your herbs is key. Lavender packs a maximum antiviral punch just as vivid blooms unfurl, waning thereafter. Echinacea stockpiles immune boosters mainly in roots in its second year. Chamomile concentrates muscle-easing compounds by mid-day when the sun is full. Each variety privately shares perfect pickup points through watched patterns.

To capture an herb's healing potential, harvest with care and timing. Rushing or getting sloppy means missing out on the supercharged compounds each plant part refines. Picking a moment too soon cuts nature's work short before the good stuff is maximized. But waiting past the peak is also wasteful; valuable properties degrade as plants dry down or fuel other processes besides wellness. There's an optimum window where potency is highest after compounds pool where your body absorbs them best.

Timing for Peak Potency

To get the most out of your homegrown medicines, pay close attention to each herb's habits. Get to know how fast different plants develop when they reach their peak, and how their prime times ebb and flow with each season. Study the signs that say, "Pick me!" for each type.

Healing compounds work on different schedules within plants. Usually, flowers and leaves are at their strongest right before blooms open, passing along peak power. Then it's the seeds' turn a few weeks later, as they finish maturing. Many plants build root potency a bit differently too. For biennials and perennials, roots bulk up over winter or their first year to power future growth. Then their root medicine levels max out in the early spring of year two. Knowing roughly when in an herb's lifetime its parts—flowers, leaves, seeds, roots—

normally reach maximum concentrations of healthy stuff helps you harvest each piece perfectly and in a timely fashion.

Recognizing Signs of Readiness

Each plant gives its signs that say, "Pick me—I'm potent!" With oregano, essential oils peak after pink bracts fade below-faded flowers as its brief window closes. Gotu kola timing is also trim-harvest, as flavorful leaf compounds focus in and before the trails of roots descend from nodes. Burdock roots slowly build defense-boosting polysaccharides over two autumns, hitting maximum size and strength just before the second winter sets in.

To master herbal medicine timing, observe your favorite healing plants closely over multiple seasons. Watch how their flowers, fruits, leaves, and roots mature and change weekly. Note harvest dates when remedies seemed most potent based on traits like taste, smell, or how easily oils were expressed. Compare notes to pinpoint each species' best plucking periods. Refine your understanding each year as your relationships with these plants deepen.

Considerations for Time of Day and Season

The sun, rain, and heat outdoors start intricate changes inside herbs daily. As conditions vary, plants make different chemicals. Timing harvests while considering these environmental cues can boost medicinal molecules to maximum levels. Whether the sun drew out oils or rain spiked potency, pay attention to each plant daily and its relationship with the world around it. Environmental impacts provide clues to catch herbal components at their healthiest heights by watching a plant's intricate responses to its growing conditions.

Many herbs, like bee balm and oregano, contain their highest essential oil concentrations mid-morning when the warming sun causes aromatic compounds to vaporize. Others, like chamomile and passionflower, accumulate more muscle-relaxing flavonoids if picked before nightfall. Still others peak twice: Mid-morning and again in late afternoon.

The season also weighs heavily; Valerian's sedative iridoids are milder in the spring but intensify through the summer heat. Skullcap's medicinal scutellarin fades as moisture and light decline into fall. Time harvests based on compound production fluxes responsive to shifting environmental stimuli.

Adjusting Harvest Times

For leaves and flowers meant to dry or be made into extracts, the best time is after the morning dew dries but before the day gets too hot, when some properties may fade. Biennial angelica roots save fewer essential oils once winter arrives, so pick in early fall to catch their peak. More delicate herbs like bee balm or basil risk mold if lingering dampness isn't fully gone by harvest, so mid-day gathering works best once all dew has evaporated. Timing harvests with each plant's nature in mind, like when Angelica's roots tail off or fragile herbs still need full sunshine, helps make the most of nature's pharmacy.

Harvesting Techniques

Harvesting medicinal herbs requires adapting techniques to the part being gathered, whether collecting leaves, flowers, ripe seeds, or digging up precious roots. Matching methods to plant structures preserves the integrity and potency of each remedy component.

Leaf Techniques

Leaves offer the most abundant ongoing harvests from herbal allies. Mastering ideal picking approaches ensures maximal flavonoids, antioxidants, and other leaf-held constituents.

Pluck leaves early in the day after dew dries but before heat or sunlight degrades delicate chemistry. Using clean scissors or pruners, cut individual leaves or whole leafy branch tips just above leaf nodes without stripping plants bare. This encourages denser, bushier regrowth.

Delicate herbs like basil need gentle handling; pick leaves individually to avoid bruising. Lay them flat to dry so nothing smushes. Heartier sage and thyme can take a bit more; grab short leafy stem sections and snip whole shoots. Bundle similar to how you'd tie flowers, standing sprigs upward so lower leaves don't get flattened as they dry. Tender and tough differ in how you harvest them. Basil wants care picking by leaf, while Sage accepts clipping its stems. Adjusting your touch protects frail botanicals better as their medicine matures further through drying.

Many herbs reward regular trimming by putting out more lush, colorful new branches. By snipping tips, plants get the message to make growth hormones that lead to bushier regrowth. But never take over a third of the shoots at a time, or the plant can't keep up. Let the bare spots refill fully before harvesting again. Strategic, frequent trims within reason cause herbs to become more abundant through triggered releafing. Light, regular pruning spurs plants to put on extra foliage for your next picking.

Flower Strategies

Flowers offer heavenly smells and special, healthy molecules. Picking them just right keeps these good things at their best. Usually, oils peak right when flowers open before plants focus on seeds. Harvest whole flower tops early, once the dew fades. Use clippers or fingers to gently snip heads into breathable containers. This prevents crushing petals as their aromas and medicine carry on providing benefits.

Certain blooms, like calendula, readily scatter seeds when bothered. To gather its potent petals for healing, pinch or snip each flower head with care, just under the bloom itself. Have a container ready below to catch any seeds ejected in the process. This allows for capturing the flower's curative power without losing its seeds to the ground. With gentle precision plucking—pinching or clipping below each calendula crown—its medicine-rich petals and seeds both stay preserved for use.

By snipping off dead blooms, you inspire herbs to keep flowering longer instead of rushing to seed. Gently pinch or trim old flower tops where they meet the leaves below, leaving behind the greenery. Be careful not to cut down too far, depriving bare stems of foliage and fueling regrowth. Do this pruning after peak blossoms to stop plants from slowing down. Regular removal of past flowers encourages new rounds to burst, extending a plant's blooming season rather than shortening its rest period.

Seed Practices

Wait until seeds are good and ripe by watching flower parts dry up and seed pods turn brown. Gently shake a few heads each day to see when the seeds feel loose. Most will spill out with just light pressure once fully mature. Don't be too hasty, though; observe the fading flowers and drying process to know the right moment. Regularly testing a few seeds prepares you for when it's prime picking time, with a little disturbance releasing them smoothly into your palm. With attentive daily checks, as ripening happens, you'll catch herbs at seed-drop perfection.

For herbs like parsley, echinacea, and mustard, cut the whole seed stalks once they're bone dry on the plant. Hang the stems upside down in breathable bags to finish drying. Give them a good shake and crush over a bucket only when fully crispy. This roughs up the prickly seed pods, freeing the seeds inside to rain down. Blow or shake off any leftover chaff and debris. Package your fresh, clean seeds in sealed containers. Properly drying and then briskly shaking loosens them with ease for trouble-free collecting and storing.

Some seeds need more care. Fragile cilantro seeds release easily just by rubbing individual dried pods between your fingers over a tray. For seeds meant to scatter in wind and weather, like mullein and amaranth, position paper or mesh under mature plants. Gently wiggle the ripening heads and let gravity do the work of collecting them below. Delicate cilantro spreads its bounty with direct, soft crumbling instead of tossing. With strategically timed shaking or hand rubbing, you can preserve even the tiniest yield for future plantings.

Root Guidelines

For herbs that come back year after year, the roots contain healing properties that strengthen as they mature. Unearth them at their best to enjoy these gifts or multiply the plants. Slide a sturdy garden fork down under the whole herb, soil, and all. Lever gently to lift without snapping the tender root structures. Use a misting hose nozzle on a light spray to rinse off any remaining dirt—no need for scrubbing. Harvesting established root systems thus preserves their potent medicinal qualities and allows them to be shared with others as plants. With careful lifting and cleansing, nutrients and growth are left intact.

Never harvest the entire root system unless lifting a plant for transplanting or collection propagation. Removing all roots kills the plant. Instead, divide mature plants, replanting a section of root mass alongside several new starts grown from seed to replace harvested specimens. This ensures a perpetual balance through seeding and root division across seasons.

Post-Harvest Care

The journey from the garden to the medicine chest continues after the harvest. Proper post-harvest handling preserves the purity, potency, and integrity of harvested home remedies. Whether promptly processing fresh herbs or carefully drying bounty for long-term storage, attention and care after gathering reward the diligent herbalist.

Gentle Handling and Cleaning

Carefully cut or pinch herbs to avoid crushing delicate leaves and flowers. Gently place them in breathable harvest baskets. Separate leaves or florets sticking together to help air circulate and prevent mold during drying. Keep harvested materials out of direct sunlight.

Speedy transport from the garden to counter limits enzymatic changes and degrading compounds. Chilled storage buys additional prep time for more delicate herbs like basil if same-day processing isn't possible. Where feasible, clean herbs in the field to reduce contamination risk.

Gently rinse herbs to remove dust, debris, and insect particles—especially important for hairy herbs like mullein and nettle. Swish leaves in cool, clean water. Allow herbs to air dry fully on towels before further processing to prohibit mold growth.

For resinous herbs like sage and thyme, skip water baths. Wiping with damp towels suffices to clean while minimizing essential oil losses from excess hydration. Discard any bruised or damaged portions that may spoil quickly. Handle herbs delicately from harvest through drying to preserve excellence.

Immediate Processing for Fresh Use

Chop or bruise leafy herbs right before adding them to vinegar, oils, or dishes to release aromatic essential oils that dissipate quickly once cut. Use mild-flavored herbs like lemon balm or mint fresh for optimal taste. Convert any leftovers into infused herbal oils or vinegar before the herbs compost.

Plants harvested at their peak potency make wonderfully effective fresh teas and tinctures. Chop herbs finely to expose more surface area for water or alcohol extraction. Cover with cool, not hot, liquid to avoid evaporating delicate, volatile compounds. Allow longer steep times, up to eight hours, for full extraction minus degradation from high heat.

Whether crafting artful culinary cuisine or home medicines, recently harvested herbs offer seasonal vitality and unmatched therapeutic power for the observant gatherer. Handle gently, process rapidly, and apply freshness to unlock nature's vibrant healing gifts.

Drying and Storage

Preserving freshly harvested herbs' healing essences relies on fastidious drying and storage methods. Managing moisture, light, and airflow minimizes degradation while retaining therapeutic chemistry within the precious plant medicines collected.

Drying Techniques for Medicinal Herbs

To help herbs keep their healing powers longer, dry them slowly in fresh air. This stops mold and rots from setting in. Bundle several leafy stems together with mini rubber bands, or lay single leaves on wire mesh shelves in a breezy spot. Every day, give the plants a little stir so all surfaces witness the winds. Where the climate cooperates with low moisture, open-air drying preserves herbs' medicinal peak. With regular, careful turning to circulate air around plant parts, their natural remedies stay safe from spoilage.

Fans can help speed things up by continually moving the air around the herbs so pockets of moisture don't get trapped. Just be careful not to blow bits of the herbs off wherever you have them laid out. A food dehydrator works well too by circulating warm air inside it. That's especially useful if you live somewhere humid since dehydrators can dry things out faster than waiting for air. The nice thing about dehydrators is that you can keep a close eye on them so the herbs don't dry out too much.

Air circulation is key, whether it is air or machine drying. High humidity gets trapped by dense herbal material, inviting mold. Keep bundles loose or layers thin for ample airflow. Turn, fluff, or stir daily to redistribute moisture release. Drying times range from a few days for leaves and flowers up to two weeks for some plump roots.

Protect potency by drying away from direct light. Wrap drying racks in cloth or paper to block light exposure, which degrades delicate plant compounds. Avoid plastic sheeting that traps rising moisture against plants. The right balance of darkness, movement, ventilation, and time retains medicinal excellence.

Proper Storage Practices

Glass jars are ideal for long-term dry herb storage. Their airtight seal, opacity, and stable composition protect the herbs from air, light, moisture, and reactive metal contamination. Dark glass offers better light protection. Clean thoroughly and ensure the jars are fully dry before filling. Other rigid containers, like food-grade plastic, work temporarily but may compromise quality over time.

Tucked away from heat, humidity, and light, thoroughly dried herbs remain vibrantly potent for a year or more. Choose dark, temperature-stable cupboard spaces away from stove and dishwasher heat and moisture. Basements or cellars offer naturally cooler, darker storage as well.

For delicate seeds, refrigeration or freezers extend their longevity for years. Place glass jars of dry seeds inside additional airtight plastic bags before chilling to prevent frost condensation from compromising storage.

Creating Herbal Preparations

Take your dried herbs and experiment with mixing them into customized teas tailored to each person's wellness needs. You can also try soaking herbs in vodka or glycerin for stronger tinctures meant for short-term issues. Those need a bit more time steeping in glass jars for a few weeks. For something soothing, gently heat carrier oils like coconut or olive oil with herbs, beeswax, and essential oils to make protective healing salves for skin irritations. It's a very rewarding experience to brew up personalized potions with your buddies while catching up.

Before your garden says "goodbye" for the winter, don't waste any leftover fresh herbs. Steep them in some vinegar or flavored oils instead. Rosemary, sage, oregano, and thyme work especially well since they have a stronger taste. Just drop the clean herbs into sterilized jars filled with good-quality vinegar or oils, making sure the herbs are fully submerged. Let them hang out on the counter, infusing for a couple of weeks. After that, strain out the herbs and transfer the now brightly colored infused liquid into some clean bottles. Come winter, you'll have these tasty and healthy elixirs to brighten up your dishes. The infused vinegar and oils will let you enjoy a little summer freshness even when the snow is falling.

Chapter 8

Making Herbal Preparations

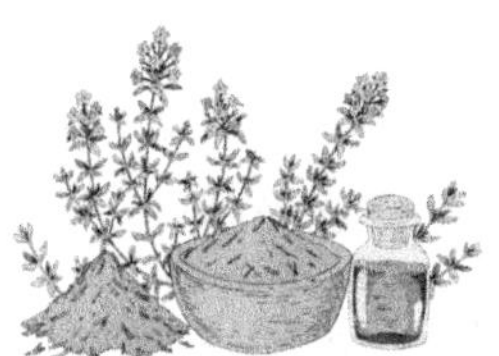

After thoughtfully nurturing medicinal herbs from seed to harvest, the final journey transforms the bundled bounty into helpful home remedies. Skillfully processing fresh or dried plant materials into usable preparations challenges the herbalist to become part alchemist and part craftsman. Through immersive hands-on practice, we begin to understand the art and science behind extracting and concentrating an herb's therapeutic gifts into convenient, consistent dosages.

While tradition gives us basic herbal directions, the true art lies in exploration. Honoring time-tested methods takes discipline, yet discovering your own pathways brings joy. Following guidelines alone leaves parts of nature's mysteries unsolved. Creativity and courage to experiment help uncover revelations waiting in plant potentials. The journey respects ancestral lore yet dares fresh steps. Both structure and wonder mentor powerful remedies from the gifts the earth bestows.

Turmeric roots infuse their potent anti-inflammatory compounds into brandy with a little help. The low heat and alcohol coax out the root's vibrant orange color and aromatic properties in a chemical-preserving way without harshly tearing the plant fibers. Meanwhile, calendula flowers share even more nourishing, skin-mending fats and oils when suspended in a carrier oil rather than water—an example of the solvent deeply impacting what medicinal compounds emerge. With strategic choices of liquid agents and temperatures, herbs generously bestow tailored wellness benefits in gorgeous, nourishing elixirs to support you inside and out.

Burdock roots lend their inulin sugars well to long, simmered tea infusions, extracting trace minerals, yet a light overnight steep preserves lemon verbena's delicate aromatic oils better. By getting our hands dirty and experimenting with various methods, we develop a feel for what each plant gives up easily and what needs coaxing. There may be some spills and waste, yet failures become lessons, and breakthroughs bring rewards. In this, we bond with nature's gifts, staining our hands with plant essences until their nuanced personalities are known.

The true miracle rests in the transformation itself, from a tiny seed to a vital healing aid through nature's graceful mystery of growth, death, and rebirth. As gardeners and caretakers, we partner imperceptibly in that poem year after year.

Principles of Extraction

Transforming harvested herbs into remedies relies on extraction—the selective transfer of plant chemicals from cellular material into a carrying solvent. Mastering foundational techniques expands an herbalist's repertoire for custom preparations.

Solvent Extraction Methods

Alcohol, vinegar, oil, and glycerin effectively pull and contain desired compounds from herbal materials through proper preparation. Each solvent solubilizes different constituents for multifaceted remedies.

Alcohol readily absorbs a wide spectrum of an herb's bioactive components, both water- and fat-soluble. The most versatile homemade menstruum, alcohol extracts enable room-temperature preservation once complete by preventing microbial growth. Popular examples are glycerites and tinctures.

Acetic acid-rich kinds of vinegar isolate different constituents, lending unique flavor and health benefits. Antimicrobial vinegars naturally resist spoilage, making them excellent solvents for mineral-rich long-term herb infusions.

Glycerin has excellent preserving qualities and sweetly highlights an herb's characteristic flavor better than alcohol or water alone. Glycerites are nice options for children and those avoiding alcohol.

Choosing the Right Solvent for Specific Herbs

To fully unlock an herb's healing talents, pair it with the right extracting liquid. Different parts of plants willingly shed their goodness into certain carriers over others. Do some homework and reference an herbal guidebook for solubility tips on what elements certain plants offer and how well they interact with various solvents. With this knowledge, you can better choose whether water, oil, alcohol, or vinegar maximizes the yield of an herb's coveted medicines. Understanding the natural attraction between botanical ingredients and their solvent suitors means crafting formulas to take full advantage of nature's gifts.

To get what you want from herbs, choose the solvent wisely. Boozy tinctures are ideal for Hawthorn berries and their bounty of flavonoids because alcohol excels at tapping alkaloids, tannins, and more. Herbs high in scents transfer smoothly into glycerin. Meanwhile, long steeps in vinegar work best for nettles and oats looking to release minerals into solution. Each herb offers hidden healing bits that favor certain carriers over others. Matching each plant's properties to a preferred liquid allows crafting preparations tuned to the intended benefits.

Water-Based Extraction

Making herbal medicines is part science and part art. For leaves, berries, and flowers and their lighter flavors, a simple steep wins their essence. Pour just-boiled water over the plant material and let it sit covered for at least 10 minutes to release the goods into solution. However, some herbs have deeper, hidden gifts that demand special treatment. Roots, bark, and fungi store wealth inside sturdy walls, needing coaxing and slow simmering over many hours. By matching steeps or decoctions to a plant's particular composition, we guide their powers while preserving fragrance and potency.

Herbal teas offer simple ways to welcome nature's blessings inside and out. Standard steeped leaf teas deliver key nutrients, minerals, and antioxidants for health. Try sunlight-steeped solar infusions, capturing light-loving compounds in clear jars. Brothy stocks extract joint-mending remedies from simmered bones and herbs. Even the skin absorbs benefits when wrapped in muslin saturated with chosen herbs. Water acts as the basic solvent for transferring healing compounds in teas, compresses, and broths.

Honoring medicinal herbs through the full cycle, from seed to helpful remedy, relies first on understanding the core principles governing extraction into personalized preparations. Lay this foundation thoughtfully, and the art of herbal alchemy unfolds in wondrous ways.

Creating Tinctures and Infusions

Herbal tinctures make it easy to access nature's remedies at any time. By steeping plants in alcohol, their concentrated healing properties are packed into a portable potion. Simple ratios and basic techniques allow for the crafting of customized healing elixirs. Take the time to learn preferred herb-to-booze mixtures and steeping methods. Then you can tailor potent preparations to meet your own unique needs or those of loved ones. Having this plant-based pharmacy on hand offers portable access to nature's pharmacy wherever life may lead.

The standard tincture formula combines:

- 1 part dried, powdered herb (1 ounce herb)
- 5 parts liquid menstruum (5 ounces solvent)

A 1:5 ratio ensures sufficient solvent fully immerses and extracts the herb material over time. Simply multiply equal ratios to make larger batch sizes as needed. Adjust the alcohol percentage to suit an herb's chemistry—at least 25% alcohol by volume—to adequately preserve it once strained (Lee, 2020).

Maceration and Percolation Techniques

Making herb tinctures at home is easy. First, cram as many dried herbs as you can fit into a glass jar, packing it to the top. Then pour your solvent, usually vodka or glycerin, right over the herbs. Give it a good stir to get rid of any air bubbles. Screw the lid on tight and give the full jar a little shake each day. Let it sit in a cool, dark place for about 4-6 weeks so the herbs have time to soak and the good stuff seeps out into the liquid. When a month has passed, it's ready to strain out the soggy herbs. Pour the now-tinctured liquid into clean bottles, and you're done! Just a bit of hands-on time is all it takes to end up with a batch of natural, DIY herbal remedies to use throughout the winter.

If you want to extract those delicious aromas from your herbs, try a slower drip method. Take a filtering basket, add your fresh or dried herbs, and put it over a container to catch the liquid below. Slowly add a small amount of your menstruum—usually vodka or glycerin—right onto the herbs so it just barely drips down into the collection vessel. Keep making slow additions until the herbs are good and saturated. Then seal it all up and let it steep for a few weeks. This gradual drip process helps preserve those volatile scent compounds. When time's up, squeeze the basket to press out the last bits of good stuff. Bottle up your nicely aromatic tincture!

Crafting Herbal Infusions

- **Tea:** This is the simplest. Just boil some water, then take your tea off the heat and add things like leaves, flowers, or berries. Give it five minutes or so to brew before drinking. The hot water draws out the tasty flavors and vitamins.
- **Decoctions:** If you're using harder plant parts like roots or bark, these need low and slow cooking. Simmer them for eight hours or more to break down the tougher material. You end up with a concentrated medicine.
- **Cold infusions:** Leave delicate fresh herbs like lemon balm in room-temperature water overnight. The long soak in cool water gently releases the good

stuff without damaging it with heat. It is great for retaining those delicate aromatic oils.

When making herbal teas, decoctions, or other extracts, it helps to know what works best for different herbs. For example, mint leaves will steep quickly in hot water and release their flavors. But something like valerian root is better suited to slow, cold soaking overnight so it doesn't lose its nice aroma compounds. Play around with the steeping times and temperatures to see what each herb prefers. You'll find some herbs like brief heating, while others need gentle handling. Take notes on your experiments so that next time you can customize the preparation method for each plant. Over time, you'll learn the best techniques for drawing out maximum taste and benefiting from your favorite herbs.

Salves, Ointments, and Creams

When making herbal skin salves, the carrier oil you choose makes a difference. Opt for quality oils that can nicely absorb the herb's helpful substances into your skin. Popular ones include olive, coconut, jojoba, almond, or apricot oil. Lighter oils, like jojoba, are better paired with more delicate herbs since they won't overpower the plant's properties. Heavier oils work well with sturdier herbs. The carrier oil acts as a soothing base that helps transfer the herb's therapeutic qualities onto your skin without over-drying. It also adds moisture and protection.

Whether you're crafting healing salves, balms, or lotions, beeswax is a wonderful natural additive. It adds a thick, creamy texture that makes the salve smoothly spreadable for comfort. Beeswax also lengthens the shelf life by helping seal out contaminants that could shorten its usability. Test different beeswax-to-oil ratios to get your desired consistency. More oil leaves it silky soft and easy to spread, but it dissipates faster. Extra beeswax firms it up into a thicker balm or even salve sticks that last longer. Go lighter on the wax if you want it softer or heavier for a more heavy-duty balm. Experiment to see what ratio works best for how you plan to use your homemade skincare.

Creating Herbal Salves for Skin Application

Homemade herbal salves are better for your skin than just using plain oils. That's because the oils can absorb into your skin while the salve protects it. To make a basic one, pick the herbs and carrier oils best for your skin type. Slowly warm the oils over a few weeks so the herbs fully soak in their benefits before straining them out. Measure the infused oil, then add about half as much beeswax. Gently melt them together until smooth, then quickly pour into containers before they set. Let it cool fully before use. From there, get creative! You can adjust recipes by using different herbs, oils, or amounts of beeswax to change the texture or customize the effects.

Crafting Ointments and Creams

You've got options beyond just herbal salves. Ointments make an extra-thick and protective rub, especially for sensitive skin areas. They use animal fat or petroleum instead of carrier oils. The process is quite similar to salve-making. Then there are antioxidant-rich whipped creams; these emulsify herbs into a blend of heated water and oil phases that get beaten together once cooled to a velvety texture. Creams allow herb properties to soak into the skin differently. No matter which you choose—salve, ointment, or cream—focus formulas on your skin's needs by researching specialized recipes online. Tailor the ingredients and preparation technique based on your skin concerns, whether it's moisturizing, healing, or anti-aging results you're after.

Making your herbal skin care last longer is easy; just boost it with some antioxidant add-ins. Rosemary extract or vitamin E oil will protect your salves as they whip up. Adding clay powders thickens things nicely too while treating your skin to minerals. Blending in essential oils fights germs and covers any herby smells from the base. When tinkering with recipes, start small at first so you can find extras that enrich the experience through scent, texture, or looks. You might stumble onto a surprise ingredient that takes your salve up a notch. Test different boosters to customize how your skincare looks, feels, and preserves the herbal benefits within.

Capsules and Powders

Herbal powders provide an easy way to enjoy plant medicine at any time. With home-fillable gelatin or veggie capsules, you can customize your own standardized herbal blends without costly machinery. By grinding botanicals to powder and pouring them into uniform-sized caps, potent doses become portable without messy teaspoons. Take supplements on the go or customize individual remedies tailored to your needs. Filling capsules offers a hands-on way to benefit from nature's pharmacy in a standard, tidy format you control. With minimal investment, you can craft individualized plant-based wellness aids.

Filling and Sealing Herbal Capsules

Filling capsules by hand takes a few basics. Pick gelatin, veggie cellulose, or HPMC caps matching how much powder fits your preferred dose. Open the halves and clamp them into a simple filling stand crafted from dowels to keep sections neatly aligned. This homemade station keeps the process organized and steady. With the right capsule size and a filler stand, you'll soon expertly pack powdered botanicals into uniform portable doses. A little trial and error unlock the satisfaction of crafting personalized plant-based supplements without a pricey gadget.

Filling capsules by hand takes practice but yields rewards. Set up over a tray for easy cleanup. Use a small funnel to heap powder into half the capsule. Gently tap the filled half against the powder container to consolidate before capping it off. To join, carefully align the bottom and top halves. Apply gentle pressure to snap them securely closed. A final twist seals the deal. With patience and a light touch, powdered plant magic becomes a portable potion. Take time to find your rhythm— messy starts pave the way for mastery.

To safely enjoy herbal supplements, do your homework on typical dosing. Use a small digital scale to weigh powders in various capsule sizes to gauge standard single portions. Consider the plant, your health goals, and your capsule's capacity when portioning out power. Clearly labeled jars let you organize blends by ingredient and creation date. Proper guidance and dosing empower well-being without worry. Trusting tradition and science helps deliver nature's wisdom reliably to nourish your unique journey.

Powdering Herbs for Consumption

Whether for supplements, cooking, or skincare, a quality herb grinder proves a handy ally. Electric models pulverize botanicals into powder quickly, sparing hands from tedious work. Adjustable settings ensure customized textures, from coarsely cut to ultra-fine, suiting any use. Burr or hammermill models efficiently power through big batches too. Thorough cleaning between plants prevents mixing flavors or compromising unique chemistries. Trusty grinders let you fully harness nature's pharmacy for body and soul with ease.

Whether sweet or savory, pulverized plants pack kitchens with therapeutic flair. Where heat might strip whole herbs of aromatic oils, grinding shares their nature-given gifts through foods and more. Spice up curry pastes, infuse teas or boost baked goods' nutrition by stirring in powders that retain potency. Their healing properties also slip effortlessly into homemade body care. Add powders to clay masks for glowing complexions or nourishing flower baths. In or out of the kitchen, reducing botanicals to fine particles spreads nature's pharmacy into daily life through versatile routes.

For swift access to herbalism's gifts, maintain a modest stock of commonly used botanicals, freshly ground. Powders unlock essence, cutting preparation. Yet watch volatile ultrafine, avoiding irritation to sensitive spots like your nose. While convenient, very fine powders may cause discomfort if inhaled directly. For your comfort, pack ultrafine powders prudently into capsules instead. Their potency stays intact, delivered gently. With care and discretion, your herbal pantry needs just a pinch of planning to spread nature's blessings wherever life may lead.

Chapter 9

Dosage and Administration of Herbal Remedies

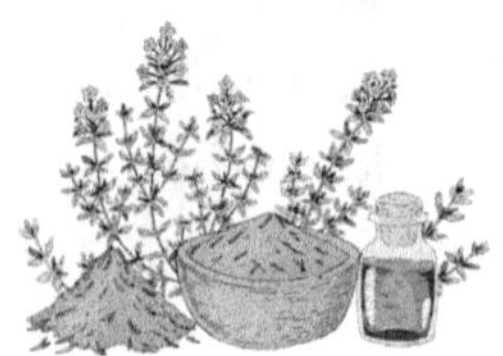

After seasons of nurturing beloved medicinal herbs from seedlings to dried bundles bursting with potent chemistry, the conscientious herbalist pauses thoughtfully before each remedy is made. We shoulder profound responsibility for bridging the divide between ancient botanical wisdom and today's unprecedented health woes. What is the safe and effective way to administer nature's healing gifts? What dosage delivers therapeutic benefits without toxicity for widely varying needs within the human mosaic?

While ancient wisdom affirms certain herbs' benefits, we approach plant medicine humbly. Biochemical processes prove intricate, so effects emerge gradually through nurturing overall wellness, not fast fixes. Traditional herbalism honors both time-tested experience and modern science's nuanced revelations. Herbs modulate bodily functions through interconnected networks, not by attack but by gentle guidance over time. Complex chronic issues rarely yield single solutions. By respecting plants' subtleties and our bodies' wisdom, herbalism's gentle nudges uphold health holistically through generations-old empirical care and cutting-edge awareness alike.

While herbs can produce powerful results, they typically do so more gently than pharmaceuticals. Their effects also take longer to kick in compared to isolated drugs. That's why herbal remedies have a good safety track record. However, plants can still impact your body and even interact with any medications you take or health issues. Traditional herbalists believe the best approach is patience: Start with low doses of one or two simple herbs and pay attention to how your body responds over time before making any adjustments. Herbs are stronger than they seem, so it's always wise to introduce them gradually into your routine. Only after you've gotten to know how your system reacts would you carefully consider tweaking the amount, duration, or specific herbs in a formula.

When it comes to herbal medicine, balancing tradition and science isn't always straightforward. On one hand, ancestral wisdom gained over centuries of people healing themselves with plants shows many herbs can be quite safe when prepared and applied appropriately. However, modern research has uncovered some hidden dangers too (De Smet, 1995). This led to it being regulated worldwide. While protecting health is important, outright bans can also restrict access to remedies that may truly help in a crisis. The truth is, that both ancestral practice and clinical findings provide pieces of the puzzle. Using a discerning approach that thoughtfully considers all available information from different knowledge lineages allows for safely benefiting from nature's pharmacy when needed most.

Determining Dosages

One cool thing about herbal medicine is that it can be tailored specifically for each person. Pharmaceuticals come with set-in-stone dosing guidelines, but herbs are more flexible. When determining how much of a remedy to take, consider three main factors: Your own health situation, the innate potency of the herb, and how concentrated the preparation method made it. Every body is different, and some herbs are naturally stronger than others. Plus, techniques like tincturing extract more of the active ingredients than a simple tea would. Take all those variables into account to dial in the right amount for your body.

Individual Factors Influencing Dosage

- **Age:** Both kids and grandparents tend to process herbal stuff a bit slower than the rest of us. It's best to start with a smaller amount if you're very young or older. Pay close attention to how your body responds before considering more.
- **Weight:** In general, heavier people may be able to handle a tad more of something than someone tiny. But everyone's different. Always test the water first with just a bit and see how it sits before increasing the dose gradually.
- **Health conditions:** If you're already taking lots of prescription medications or dealing with ongoing health issues, adding herbs to the mix deserves some extra careful thought. Your body is going through a lot as it is. Talk to your doctor first, so they're in the loop.

Recognizing the Potency of Different Herbs

Certain herbs are seriously potent; it's amazing just how little you need to feel an effect. Herbs like evening primrose, damiana, and wild yam contain substances that influence your hormones, so you'll notice their impact. Only a tiny, infrequent dose is required from these intensely active plants. While they may seem mild, these herbs demand respect for how strongly they can interact with your body's delicate systems. It's always best when using very potent herbs to do so under the guidance of an experienced herbalist. They understand your full medical history and can help ensure you use powerful botanicals safely in small amounts, carefully monitored over time.

When trying out an herb for the first time, especially one with undefined potency, go slow. Even if a plant is considered generally safe, each person reacts differently. Your body is unique. Don't assume that because others tolerate higher amounts, your body will too. Some herbs are inconsistent from crop to crop in their active levels, so you need that buffer.

General Dosage Guidelines

To safely test an herb's benefits, look to vetted plant medicine guides and practitioners for typical starting doses. Think of these as breadcrumb suggestions, not strict laws—guiding lights to shape initial trials toward therapeutic outcomes. Bodies differ, and herbs affect us uniquely. So, dosages serve to point us down pathways, not lock us rigidly onto pre-set courses. Experts' parameters, not declarations, empower thoughtful self-care within nature's pharmacy for those curious yet cautious souls.

Experienced herbal practitioners gain insight, allowing deeper customization. Through attentive intake discussions exploring clients' individual issues and backgrounds, they craft tailored herbal strategies. These experts finely adjust specific plants, amounts, and schedules to complement each person. Where generalized starting points serve as orientation, herbalists' personalized care steers remedies with a stronger footing. By grasping complex root causes and sensitively targeting wellness from within, their guided fine-tuning empowers greater relief through nature's pharmacy.

The way an herb is prepared and taken makes a big difference in how strong it is and how long it works. For example, if taking it in capsule form, the dosage is usually between 0.3-6 grams per day (Watts, n.d.) (Basicmedicalkey Admin, 2016). If using a tincture, the daily amount is normally 30–60 drops (WishGarden Herbs, 2012). For teas, the typical dosage is steeping 1-4 grams of the dried herb in a cup of hot water. It's important to pay attention to these differences between preparations because how concentrated or diluted an herb is impacts how much you need to take to get the potential benefits. Always check the recommendations for the specific product or formula you are using.

Methods of Administration

The easiest way to benefit from herbs is to drink them as teas or take them in tinctures, capsules, or your regular foods and beverages. This allows you to control the dosage yourself for mild daily support up to strong antimicrobial effects. However, it's important to properly prepare the herbs for oral consumption to ensure both safety and effectiveness. Be sure to follow instructions for steeping, extraction, or formulation to reap the rewards while avoiding any potential side effects.

- **Tinctures:** Tinctures are a handy way to get a bunch of plant goodness into your body. Use an eyedropper to measure out 30-60 drops of the herbal alcohol mix (WishGarden Herbs, 2012); shake it up first. Feel free to add a splash of water if it's strongly flavored.

- **Teas**: Steeping dried plants in hot water is relaxing and provides hydration and healing benefits. Try steeping about one teaspoon of herb per cup for a healthy drink. Extend the steeping time or add more tea to alter the strength.

- **Infusions:** Long infusions where you soak herbs overnight really saturate the water with minerals, natural sugars, and alkaloids. Follow a recipe you trust as a starting point, then adjust to your preference.

Start low and go slow when determining the ideal oral doses for new herbs. Keep intake records detailing preparation specifics, dosage times or amounts, and perceived effects or side effects. Gradually increase the dosage every three to seven days if there are no noticeable benefits to reach satisfying results. Adjust again if you are ill.

Topical Application

Rubbing herbal oils, salves, and lotions onto your skin can treat surface-level issues while also delivering the plant compounds deeper through your dermal layers and into blood circulation. As absorption through the skin happens slowly at low levels, there are minimal concerns about side effects. You can use topical herbal remedies infrequently without much worry. Applying herbal formulations to your skin opens up an easy way to access some of nature's healing benefits from herbs in a convenient and generally quite safe manner.

Herbal creams are great for moisturizing your skin and also delivering oil- and water-soluble plant compounds to problem spots. Thicker salves and ointments are especially good for protecting wounds while promoting healing; choose the consistency that matches your skin's needs. When applying to wounds, lightly apply the herbal preparation just below and move outwards from the opening rather than directly into it. This helps push any infection away rather than trapping it inside. Reapply two to three times per day or as needed once the previous application has been fully absorbed.

Since different herbs, formulations, and skin conditions all impact absorption in their own way, there aren't strict rules for how much topical herbal remedy to use. The best approach is to gently apply enough to cover the problem area without creating a thick layer that could block airflow to healing wounds. Keep an eye out for any rashes, swelling, or discomfort after using a topical remedy; if that happens, wash the area and take a break from using that product. It's always a good idea to consult your doctor as well, just in case. You can potentially retry using a very diluted version later on, but listen to your body's feedback on what works best for your unique situation.

Inhalation and Aromatherapy

Inhaling herbal aromas from gentle heating methods or room diffusers allows active oil compounds to be quickly absorbed through your lung tissues and into blood circulation. There's also a psychological piece: More traditional methods like factory production seemed to enhance desired effects more. In terms of dosing with inhaled oils, it comes down to the number and length of breaths taken of the vapors. When trying a new essential oil, go slowly at first to see how your body responds.

Start with just a few short breaths and increase from there as you become familiar with how a particular oil affects you.

When inhaling essential oils, be aware that the membranes in your nose and lungs can be easily overwhelmed. It's best to diffuse the oils for short 10-minute bursts in a well-ventilated, large room rather than continuously in small, enclosed spaces. Also, pay attention to how individual herbs might affect your lungs; inhaling leaves and flowers is generally gentle, but resins, roots, camphor, menthol, or eucalyptus could potentially irritate sensitive respiratory tissue. If you find an oil irritating when inhaled, switch to applying it diluted in a thick cream or salve on your skin instead, as this delivery method puts less stress on the lungs.

The way you take herbal medicine matters since it affects the dosage your body receives. Preparations like internal tinctures or external salves introduce herbs into your system in a slower, more gradual way compared to isolates in capsules or pills. This gives you—as the home healthcare provider—more control over dosing and the chance to adjust based on how your body reacts. You can pay attention to hints from your plant allies about what works best for you as an individual. Plus, you'll notice personal responses over multiple uses, allowing tweaks as needed. Methods involving digestion or application to the skin provide a flexible approach, so you can build up tolerance thoughtfully by staying tuned in to subtle feedback.

Tracking and Adjusting Treatment

Paying attention to small shifts in your body is so important when taking herbal medicines. Keeping a journal of your herbal journey lets you track what's working and what could use adjusting. Be sure to write down specifics for anything you take:

The herb or combo, the brand or batch, how much in what form (tea, tincture, and so on), when and how often it was dosed, and how it was prepared. Note any effects felt, positive or negative. Also include lifestyle stuff that could influence results, like your diet or activities. With accurate records, you can spot patterns to fine-tune your herbal protocol over time based on what real-world experience shows truly helps your unique situation.

When journaling your herbal remedies, be detailed yet consistent so it's easy to spot any shifts. Jot down how you're feeling one to two times each day, using the same words and rating scale. Note the effects shortly after dosing and again the next morning. Be sure to cover what the herbs are targeting, like sleep, mood, digestion, pain levels, and more. Don't forget to list what you eat, how active you are, stress changes, or if you have altered any medications—all of which can impact results. Taking just a few minutes to carefully log symptoms, foods, and lifestyle factors will make it simple to analyze over time if an herb is working for your situation or if tweaks may be needed.

Over weeks, patterns should emerge revealing effective dosing levels and schedules.

With herbal medicine, you want to see that things are gradually headed in the right direction. Little improvements to your energy, pain levels, or sleep quality are signs a remedy may be a good match. If, after two weeks, you notice benefits but have room for more, it's okay to raise the dosage a tad at a time up to the maximum recommended amount. However, if nothing seems to change after two weeks at the current dose, it may be worth trying a different herb or blending in a second one to give your body a boost. And if maximum dosing still isn't giving results, talk to an expert herbalist; they can help determine if you need an alternative prescription or if another approach entirely could be better.

Equally important to track are any side effects from herbal remedies, like tummy troubles, headaches, dizziness, or worsening pain. If minor issues pop up, consider lowering the dose or how often you take it to see if that helps. If severe symptoms arise, such as difficulty breathing or swelling, stop using the herb right away. Your health and safety come first. It's also wise at that point to see a medical professional. They can help determine if an underlying condition could be exacerbated or if an allergy exists.

Consulting Healthcare Providers

While herbal medicine safely supports health for many, working respectfully with licensed providers maximizes care. Especially when addressing complex issues, the collaborative discussion identifies safe botanical integration alongside standard approaches.

Herbs empower people, reclaiming authority within the healing process without abandoning scientific advances. Responsible integration utilizes the best of both models—honoring innate healing wisdom while allowing technological gifts.

Inform all care providers of the supplements used so they may consider potential interactions with prescribed therapies. Ask for oversight when introducing new herbs if you are taking multiple medications or you are unsure of their appropriateness for your current health state. Established herbalists help navigate revegetating terrain.

Open Communication with Healthcare Professionals

Recognize that most conventional practitioners receive little botanical education. Constructive conversations build mutual understanding, enhancing their ability to support patients incorporating herbs. Share observed benefits from herbal interventions, reputable information on botanical disease treatments, and offers to log remedies tried.

Give early doubts or dismissals of non-pharmaceutical choices some leeway, as they are often excluded. Sustaining courteous exchanges fosters openness; abrupt shifts in attitude are uncommon.

Recognizing Red Flags

While most herbs gently shore wellness, certain symptoms indicate the need for urgent medical rulings and home remedies. Severe reactions like shortness of breath, dangerously low blood pressure, liver pain, or drug-like neurological symptoms deserve immediate medical evaluation. Track minor digestive or skin sensitivity for trends warranting guidance.

Those new to herbalism minimize risk through mentorship from an experienced herbal clinician well-versed in materia medica. They personalize combinations and dosing to health histories while monitoring effects until personal precision develops. Later, their wisdom steadies independent farmers along with the lifelong plant-human collaboration.

Honoring all pathways supporting vibrant well-being, we thoughtfully tend the intersections joining modern and traditional healing streams on this winding journey toward wholeness.

Chapter 10

Creating Personalized Herbal Regimens

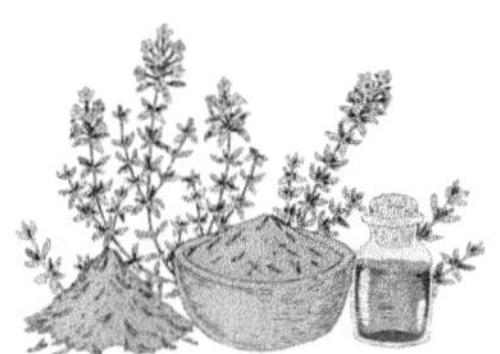

Like an artist thoughtfully mixing paints on a canvas, the skilled herbalist artfully blends botanical brushes to restore health's vibrant image. Beyond standard formulas, personalized precision treatment selects ideal remedies matching individual imbalance patterns, lifestyles, and genetic heritage for optimal resonance.

Healing isn't just about throwing chemicals at the problem to force the body to fix itself. True wellness doesn't come from an analytical, mechanical approach either. Healing springs from nurturing the innate wisdom within each of us. A skilled herbalist or health practitioner acts as a compassionate mirror, thoughtfully supporting each individual to remember and reconnect with their own inner guide. Customized care addresses both a person's unique make-up as well as the specific disease process they're facing. The goal isn't to jam repairs through willpower alone but rather to empower self-healing through gentle reflection tailored to the whole unique being—body, mind, and spirit.

The Green Glow

Healing works best when it brings all the divided parts of ourselves back into harmony. A good healer acts like a soothing salve, seeping deep where it's needed—into the places within us that have dried up under illness or been left behind due to loneliness and disconnection from who we truly are. At their best, such companions gently reintroduce us to our buried essence and nature, just as remedies can renew forgotten aspects of our being. Skillful help simply reacquaints us with our own deepest resources and truth.

Caring guidance can gently illuminate the path forward through thoughtfully sharing healing tales and histories, offering a companion simply beside each unique traveler until their inner wisdom softly reawakens. Deeper questions consider which herbs, preparations, nutritious sustainers, periods of rest, and social connections might best unlock formerly frozen places holding hidden wholeness captive. But the answers to restoring flow where stiffness has set in don't come from external lists alone. The remedies are already quietly calling within in a language more ancient than the plants themselves if only we remembered how to listen with the ears of our spirit once more.

When general recommendations don't do the trick, thoughtful listening and personalized herbal blends can help find alternative routes back to healing. The most skilled practitioners closely observe each person's unique reactions to different herbal formulations. Through these subtle cues that generic guidelines may overlook, reliable care emerges tailored to the individual. By bearing gentle witness to the innate responses, an intuitive herbalist can discern which preparation truly resonates and guide the body back to balance.

Assessing Individual Health Needs

The most insightful herbalists don't just look at health issues in detached isolation; they see the whole person. Through compassionate discussions, they work to uncover the complex web of habits, relationships, and routines that underlie well-being—the supporting factors as well as areas ripe for improvement. Good herbal medicine considers emotional, mental, and social elements alongside physical ones. A skilled practitioner evaluates wellness by gently exploring all the interconnected pieces that influence how fully we can thrive, not just diagnosing symptoms separately but understanding what truly nourishes or hinders overall balance.

Begin With Questions

When assessing well-being, explore multiple important lifestyle aspects. How do you generally nourish your body—what do you eat, how active are you, and how do you recharge? It's also useful to reflect on how you process emotions and handle life's pressures. Beyond physical habits, meaningful social connections and one's mental outlook significantly impact health. Additionally, the environments we spend time in and how we're exposed to different influences can either support or deplete our energy reserves over time. Our genetic backgrounds also play a role, granting both strengths and innate sensitivities.

Distinguish between recent issues and more deeply ingrained patterns that have developed over many years. This could include physical habits like posture and dietary practices, as well as underlying thoughts and beliefs that have been adopted as ways of coping. It's useful to take a holistic look back over their entire lifetime, considering how their experiences have shaped factors like stress levels, injuries, turning points, and available supports systemically throughout their body and mind. This broader view helps identify not only sources of tension and guarding but also glimmers of resilience that hint at optimism struggling to emerge despite challenges.

Identifying Specific Health Goals and Challenges

When starting herbal medicine, define clearly what better looks like for your particular health goals. What specific areas like heart, gut, pain levels, mood, or energy need help, and in what timeline would incremental gains seem achievable? Outlining the vitality destination you're aiming for keeps you focused. It also lets you periodically check that you're on track toward meeting reasonable benchmarks. Be mindful of stalls too; look for potential hurdles getting in the way, like stress, poor sleep, or dietary habits that may warrant addressing. Having a clear picture makes it easy to monitor if remedies are truly moving the needle and reveal when tweaks may light a fire under progress.

It's worth asking ourselves: What old ideas, no longer serving us well, do we cling to without realizing? Past hurts or harsh self-talk can unconsciously hold us back from full wellness more than dysfunctional genes alone. When we heal within, letting go of outdated, limiting views formed during low points, our body often follows suit. Transforming fixed beliefs that wrongly defined us through temporary struggles opens the door to bigger change. Physical states don't dictate our true selves; we all deserve to rediscover our natural, vibrant essence without restraints from the past.

Individual Factors Influencing Herbal Choices

When considering herbs for kids and seniors, it's smart to factor in more than just age. For example, elderberry is generally fine for supporting a young immune system but could stir up too much inflammation for someone already fighting off illness. Meanwhile, relaxing passionflower soothes anxious minds yet might overly fatigue elders seeking uplift versus calm. Tailoring herbal choices and dosages to individual needs offers a wiser approach. A youth facing stress or an elder battling infection likely benefits differently than their unencumbered peers.

Blending Herbs for Synergistic Effects

Experienced herbalists have a real knack for crafting custom blends that highlight each plant's special qualities. They understand the energetic essence of different herbs and carefully choose combinations to magnify healing goals while minimizing potential issues. Watching a skilled formulator at work is like witnessing a jazz great improvise. They take the unique energies of solo herbs and weave them together harmoniously into a personalized melange greater than any ingredient alone. Where mainstream medicine sees only chemistry, these clinicians perceive subtle synergies to shape just the right botanical symphony tailored for each patient.

Our bodies often have natural tendencies to feel damp, dry, or like we run hot or cold, depending partly on the weather and seasons. With a bit of self-observation, you can determine your own constitutional type, and choosing complimentary herbs can help balance things out. Those with fiery, high-energy natures will find peppermint and its cousins soothing. Meanwhile, people prone to dry skin or hair will appreciate the moisture-boosting benefits of mildly softening roots. Tailoring your herbal routine to your particular make-up, whether influenced by genetics or current climate conditions, ensures you select allies that work naturally with your system instead of against it.

Some herbs just seem meant to work together and get results. For example, black pepper makes turmeric's anti-inflammatory power more bioavailable. Meanwhile, a little fat enhances your body's absorption of cannabis compounds. Licorice also helps respiratory remedies like cough syrups penetrate the lungs better. With experience, an herbalist learns the smart ways to combine allies so their positive effects multiply. Harmonizing herbs based on how their subtleties align maximizes healing potential for the mind, body, and spirit.

Herbal Combinations for Specific Goals

Combining herbs for relaxation and stress reduction:

Bliss Blend

Try this soothing herbal tea recipe for relaxation, called *bliss blend*. It combines herbs well-known for their calming properties. Use one part skullcap, which helps soothe anxious feelings and ease tension throughout the body. Add a half part passionflower to promote restful sleep. Finally, include a quarter part hawthorn berry to center and calm the heart. Steep this trio of stress-easing botanicals in hot water, then cozy up and unwind with a calming cup of herbal medicine from nature's pharmacy. The blend honors each plant's properties to relieve anxiety, aid slumber, and relax the entire mind and body.

Creating blends for immune support and overall well-being:

Whole Health Elixir

Boost your immunity and overall well-being with this versatile herbal blend called *whole health elixir*. It adds Astragalus, a famous tonic herb that supports the immune system. Add in

Ashwagandha, which reduces stress levels by nourishing the adrenals. To aid circulation, add ginger rhizome. Then, include a touch of cayenne for its metabolism-revving properties. With two parts each of Astragalus and Ashwagandha as the base, then one part ginger and a quarter part spicy cayenne. It makes a refreshing tea to keep your body running at its best through the cold and flu season or anytime you want to give your health a healthy lift in a single cup.

Skillfully mingling complementary herbs based on energetic themes fine-tunes formulas for efficacy on all levels of well-being.

Regimens for Common Conditions

Respiratory Health

Keeping your breathing clear during seasons when colds and allergies strike requires a wise approach. Your herbal protocol needs balancing immune support without potential overstimulation. Custom herbal remedies for respiratory wellness gently prepare your defenses against intruders without excessively fueling reactions. Thoughtful combinations of herbs that boost immunity yet soothe inflammation reduce the risk of issues like coughs dragging on. By mindfully matching plants to your body's current needs, you can stay healthy through changes in weather and exposure to bugs.

When a cough strikes, it's your lungs working hard to keep you healthy. Coughing helps expel irritants and germs that could do damage. The best herbal remedies for coughing ease the throat and chest just enough to make clearing phlegm a breeze without hindering this important defense process. You want to gently soothe inflamed tissues so coughs aren't uncomfortable.

Bronchitis Cough Syrup

Relieve your troublesome cough with this herbal syrup. Use thyme and elderberry to lend antimicrobial power against chest infections. Wild cherry bark sedates the cough reflex for relief without full suppression. Licorice root, a longtime respiratory tonic, adds further support. And honey coats and soothes the throat. Try one teaspoon, as needed for wet or dry coughs, up to four times a day. Adjust the herbs inside to your tastes; thyme or licorice could stand out more based on your needs. Experiment with this versatile remedy to quiet coughs and give your lungs the care they call for during congested times.

Seasonal Allergy Formula

For seasonal allergies, finding relief involves lowering inflammation at various stages instead of just one. This herbal formula tackles multiple aspects of the irritating chain reaction. Stinging nettle is a natural antihistamine. Butterbur extract blocks leukotrienes and their sneeze-inducing effects. Quercetin, paired with bromelain from pineapple, helps stabilize overreactive mast cells. Local bee pollen may also aid in building tolerance over time. Try taking this combination 10–14 days before allergy season hits and intermittently during exposure periods. Addressing different reaction components holistically better supports your body through unpredictable pollen shifts that cause watery eyes and sniffles year after year.

For ongoing protection against seasonal bugs and allergens, consistently take adaptogenic herbs that strengthen your resilience. Gentle tonics like astragalus root, thyme leaf, and reishi mushroom in a daily tea go below the surface to bolster your mucosal immunity over the long haul. They support a balanced immune response without causing overreactions that lead to more issues. Rather than firefighting acute symptoms, build your underlying defenses gradually with adaptogens that help prevent intruders from getting a foothold.

Digestive Health

Taking good care of your gut over the long run requires a tailored approach. Eating nourishing whole foods, managing stress, and supporting your digestive bacteria are all important. But gentle herbal medicine can also play a key role when digestive issues strike. The right herbal remedy works with your body's specific needs, whether it's gas, bloating, constipation, or another concern. By understanding how foods, lifestyle habits, and specific botanicals interact with your individual assimilation challenges, you can restore balance and promote continued digestive well-being for life.

Indigestion Formula

Sooth occasional tummy troubles with this herbal blend for indigestion. Use fennel seed to ease gas and bloating. Ginger root revitalizes the digestive process. And meadowsweet offers protective coating support. Prepare and consume one cup of tea a full 20 minutes before eating, depending on your usual symptoms and meal size. Let your specific signs, like discomfort, gas, or acidity, guide how many herbs work best. This formula taps nature's pharmacy to alleviate digestive irregularities by addressing the issues through gentle botanical allies.

Constipation Relief

Need occasional constipation relief? Try this nighttime herbal tea that will have you feeling lighter by morning. Steep half a Senna pod for 10 minutes to provide eliminative stimulation overnight. Add one teaspoon each of Triphala powder, an ayurvedic bowel tonic, and Slippery Elm bark powder, which softens and soothes the digestive tract. Drinking this herbal concoction before bed will encourage things to move along smoothly by daybreak. While effective temporarily, focus on rebalancing your routine with enough water, fiber, and activity for long-term digestive regularity. This formula offers natural assistance without dependence when occasional irregularities strike.

Taking good care of your gut every day involves nourishing your digestive bacteria and supporting natural function. Eat prebiotic foods and take demulcent herbs like marshmallow and oat straw to coat and comfort your GI tract. Opt for gluta-mine-rich proteins to seal tissues. Add nervine herbs like chamomile and lemon balm to ease stomach stress and tension. Incorporate balancing bitters like dandelion root to stimulate your GI glands and boost digestion. Burdock root delivers detox support too. These mild botanicals work with your body to allow nutrients to be absorbed properly. Don't forget fermented foods to feed your friendly gut flora as well. With your digestive bacteria, cells, and secretions well supported, your gut health can thrive each day.

Stress and Anxiety

Overactivation of our innate fight-or-flight response due to an unbalanced neurological system takes life force energy and promotes inflammation and illness. Herbal nervines helps you cope with life's obstacles more gracefully by restoring a balanced stress response.

Nerve Nourishing Formula

If stress has you feeling fried, this herbal blend can help nourish frazzled nerves. The nerve-nourishing formula combines lemon balm, an adaptogenic stress reliever, with hawthorn leaf and flower to support your heart during tense times. The skullcap helps ease overall nervous tension. Take the tincture midday and at bedtime to hydrate nerves worn thin by constant worry or reactivity. Over time, it may undo the buildup of recurring anxious feelings better left in the past. For quick relaxation on bad days, carry rescue inhalers or buy the tincture in a smaller dropper bottle for relief anytime anxiety strikes. These natural helpers aim to soothe the mind and spirit when life gets chaotic.

Managing stress levels in a long-lasting way means making deeper changes, not just looking for quick fixes. Certain herbs and foods may help retrain your body to respond to stressors more calmly over time. Natural options like ashwagandha, rhodiola, holy basil tea, cordyceps mushroom, and reishi mushroom promote more flexibility in your adrenal glands and stress hormone production. By incorporating small amounts of these into your daily routine, you can establish healthier rhythms between when your body needs to be alert or at rest. The key is going slow—start with low doses and gradually increase over several weeks. Pay attention to how different stressors in your life affect you and focus on treatment there first. With patience and consistency, you should start to feel your stress response is under better control without unwanted side effects like being hyper or crashing.

Sleep Support

Certain herbs can softly help your body unwind and get better-quality sleep when you're feeling stressed or having trouble shutting your mind off at night. Establishing a relaxing pre-bed routine and using strategic herbal teas and supplements only as needed work together gently over time. Making time for calming activities before bed trains your internal clock to associate night with rest.

Herbal Bedtime Routines for Better Sleep

If you struggle with sleep, creating a calm pre-bed routine with soothing herbal teas can help your body unwind and prepare for better-quality rest. Around 45 minutes before bedtime, try steeping a relaxing blend of chamomile for relaxation, passionflower to promote extended sleep, valerian root for sedation, and lemon balm to quiet the busy mind. You can also enhance this nightly routine with an Epsom salt bath, which absorbs quickly to reduce physical tension. Follow with a magnesium-rich lotion massage; both bath and lotion help escalate the relaxing effects. Round it out by diffusing a few drops of calming lavender essential oil near your bed, allowing its fragrance to further embody the transition toward restful stillness.

Middle of the Night Restoration Blend

If you sometimes find yourself waking in the middle of the night and having trouble falling back asleep, a restorative herbal blend can gently soothe your nervous system and encourage more rest. Try mixing skullcap to calm the nerves, passionflower to relax the mind, and hops for sedation into a small glass of warm nut milk. You can sip up to three times through the night as needed for resets without feeling groggy in the morning. This targeted formula uses mild botanicals to rescue unwelcome waking episodes. Apply it topically as well for a lighter effect.

Chapter 11

Building a Community Around Herbal Medicine

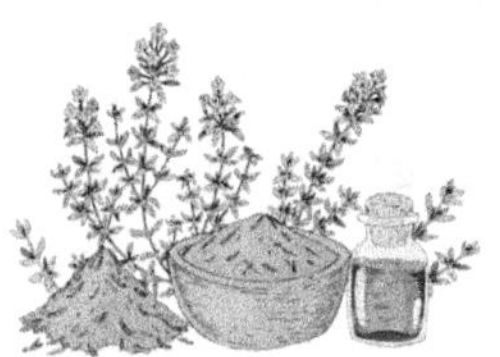

While working with herbs individually can deeply benefit your wellness journey, connecting with others who share a passion for plants also fosters positive change. Joining a community centered around herbalism does more than simply allow for the exchange of remedy tips or discussions of botanical properties. Witnessing each other's paths to greater well-being and supporting each other through both challenges and triumphs is what truly connects people. With compassion, we recognize our common humanity. By coming together vulnerably and bearing compassionate witness to healing processes, bonds are formed that nurture holistic growth beyond any single person's experience.

Getting a new perspective from others can help enrich your wellness journey, just as compost invigorates tired soil. Outside opinions shed light on unnoticed habits or beliefs that may inadvertently hold you back. With caring support that normalizes the ups and downs, feedback from trusted sources then fertilizes new insights and moves you past limiting mindsets.

Healing is a process that rarely follows a straight path, just as nature's rhythms ebb and flow across seasons. Like a midwife ensures safe birthing through challenges, an herbalist's role is to foster steady progress, reminding us that storms too shall pass and our innate drive to blossom will eventually see us through to deeper thriving on the other side.

When people come together to explore plant medicines, it has a way of bringing hidden thoughts and feelings to the surface in a supportive group setting. Sharing life's difficulties with others who understand them creates an opportunity for personal growth and shared wisdom. Oftentimes, what we perceive as individual problems are parts of a larger human experience. Connecting with our true selves helps weave separate threads into a tapestry of community strength and healing. Through openness, old wounds find renewal.

When pursuing herbal healing, approach other practices and cultures with empathy, respect, and care for proper context. Simply acquiring remedy recipes without understanding their traditions risks unintended harm. Lasting knowledge emerges from genuine relationships, not superficial extraction. By humbly learning within established frameworks as a welcomed participant rather than claiming a right to proprietary knowledge, the deeper meaning is revealed over time. The plants will share their secrets when one seeks to understand them rather than just acquire them.

Local and Online Herbal Communities

Beyond digital realms, local herbal communities gift profound healing through in-person communal rituals, hands-on knowledge sharing, nature immersions, and heart-to-heart support for nurturing well-being.

Seek out professional clinical herbalists offering plant-focused wellness consultations or apprenticeships. Attend seasonal wildcrafting tours, harvesting favored medicinal plants. Volunteer propagating or gardening at nurseries to expand regional herbal abundance. Investigate apothecaries, herb schools, craft workshops, native plant groups, community acupuncture clinics, and holistic centers hosting introductory classes or open herb walks to build plant-ally relations.

Join or Form Community Herbalism Clubs

Gather friends for regular herb exploration. Share tea while creating raised garden beds for neighborhood healing plants or cleaning up children's park spaces for accessible harvest zones. Volunteer your natural plant knowledge to support school science classes. Swap herbal ideas, elder interviews, or weed walk discoveries. Distill precious experiences into zines or blogs, amplifying unheard voices. Let purpose and structure arise organically through participant co-creation.

Online Herbal Forums and Platforms

Virtual conversations supplement the local community, opening access to global perspectives while building relationships and clinical confidence.

Introduce yourself to established professional herbal forums to discuss materia medica, clinical questions, ethical sourcing, or legal considerations with seasoned colleagues and trained clinicians worldwide. Search podcast archives on favorite herbs or challenges for mentor wisdom supporting independent study.

Hashtag searches provide extensive inspiration for platform searches. Follow or join groups dedicated to medicinal plants, ethical wild harvesting, herbal product business support, and

clinical therapy advice to enjoy daily idea exchanges and cama-
raderie.

Integrate offline and online opportunities for well-rounded,
diverse plant communion. Value deep presence while gently
reducing digital consumption. Maintain equitable inclusion
while maintaining complexity. Though imperfect, collective
wisdom propels missions of healing justice forward together.

Share Knowledge and Resources

While formal institutional frameworks undoubtedly contribute
valuable clinical herbal discoveries, informal exchanges of
direct experience hold equal weight in validating grassroots
healing traditions persisting through centuries of cultural
disruption.

Share Personal Experiences and Insights

Make space for marginalized voices through courageous listen-
ing. Seek out respected village elders who are still seed-keeping
regional plant knowledge. Show up open-hearted to testimony
from all persons living in interdependence with plants, soils,
and places in deep intimacy through blood memory and innate
sensibilities refined over generations of reciprocal service
through crisis and celebration.

Set aside assumptions that oral traditions lack sophistication
compared to peer-reviewed journals. Make allies anywhere
your relative degree of privilege allows, collectively mapping
the vibrant terroir of botanical relatives and human healers who
tend them within regional bioregions.

Participate respectfully in ethical, decolonized research initia-
tives guided by Indigenous values and incorporating commu-

nity feedback mechanisms. Offer skills strengthening localized food and medicine autonomy—seed saving, land restoration, botanical sanctuary establishment, youth education, and so on. Follow the guidance on wise action from frontline voices most impacted by historical injustices.

Herbal Resource Libraries

Volunteer to organize community seed libraries, pollinator gardens, teaching kitchens, reading rooms, medicine-making workshops, or clinics providing inclusive hands-on herbal service opportunities outside elite institutions. Regular public work parties keep projects accessible.

Help build, manage, and utilize transparent communal platforms like ethical foraging apps tracing abundance zones or collaborative herb chemical and medical action databases crowdsourcing global contributions. Ensure information access for those needing it most while mindfully considering digital divides.

Uplift collective knowledge generated through communal effort and care. Stay curious about intersectional environmental justice. Keep showing up!

Ethical Wildcrafting

Connecting with plants through respectful wildcrafting can create a deep bond that is missed when using only commercially grown herbs. However, be realistic in your approach. Fragile urban or public green spaces may not always sustain harvesting. Nature reserves require care, not just taking. Feelings of oneness are fine, but don't let romanticism replace responsibility. Thriving wilderness needs active protection too. When wild gathering, make sure populations remain intact where you collect by rotating plant parts used over time. Stewarding the land preserves its gifts for generations of appreciative herbalists, so only harvest where growth is truly abundant through natural or nurtured means.

To forage sustainably, blend ancestral practices with today's awareness. Harvest only common, hardy plants at their peak when seeds have spread, allowing continued abundance. Learn each plant as an individual, but also its role within the larger landscape, to maintain ecosystems through change. Say "thanks" for nature's gifts and offer small tokens of gratitude, completing the cycle of give-and-take. Wise elders passed knowledge enabling natural balance; we uphold those lessons with modern respect. Knowing interconnections lets land stay fruitful for all.

Help conserve biodiversity through thoughtful choices. Source from small growers who nurture endangered local plants saved from development. Become stewards yourselves by caring for overlooked areas like abandoned ravines. Nurture native plants through reseeding and pulling invasive species during volunteer work days. Look to age-old land management practices like controlled burns, coppicing trees, and using grazing animals, which flourished alongside certain flora before being displaced. With diligent, long-term care of untamed spaces through natural techniques, delicate plants will thrive once more as indicators of a restored ecosystem balance. Our lands benefit when communities actively protect declining natural riches together.

Bring nature back into your community by organizing casual plant walks with neighbors. Teach each other how to properly identify and gather information from overlooked, edible, and healing species that thrive unexpectedly around town. Chart where weedy areas, railroad lands, and alleyways harbor nourishing remnants from the past or new migrants sprouting from disrupted earth. Researching these places' forgotten cultural heritage adds depth to spotting nature's surprises. Rediscovering natural treasures hidden in plain sight is rewarding. Your neighborhood becomes more vibrant as you appreciate the resilient plants quietly supporting health, history, and habitat amid the concrete.

Lend a helping hand to overlooked areas positively impacting people's well-being outside of corporate farming. Respectfully shine a light on how marginalized green spaces in cities still provide food security for humans or wildlife. Create nonprofit harvest share programs channeling wild plants to clinics serving uninsured patients, food banks offering culturally significant ingredients, and environmental groups restoring Indigenous ties to the earth. Through thoughtful sharing of nature's gifts, undervalued domains gain appreciation while community members obtain traditional medicines and foods. When we support diverse models of land stewardship outside mainstream control, both people and the planet can benefit from more sustainable and just relationships with the land, nourishing us all.

Conclusion

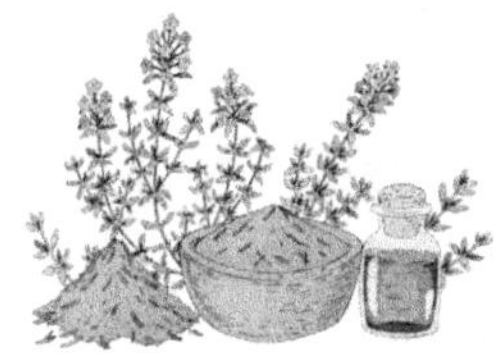

Growing your herbs and making remedies seems daunting at first. But gradually, through doing and learning, it starts clicking in a fulfilling way. Remember how much you've taken in so far—the core ideas and techniques are there inside you now. That inner wealth means cultivating vibrant gardens and crafting helpful remedies that are within your grasp to experience for yourself. The more you nurture nature's gifts with your hands, the more intuitive they will become. There's always room to learn more. For now though, you have the basic tools to begin this journey and watch your confidence blossom alongside the herbs!

Think back on all you've explored within these pages. From ancient wisdom to modern-day care, I hope sharing this herbal bouquet has given you a full, balanced understanding. Knowing plants' roles throughout history helps in choosing companions for your well-being. Now your green oasis can bloom wherever you are. A customized layout leaves space to experiment as your journey grows. How wonderful to have these living lessons take root, with the flexibility to reshape each year alongside your learning.

Getting started with essentials like beginning seeds indoors, relocating small plants in the ground, multiplying existing herbs, and taking regular care makes sure your garden grows strong. Addressing any issues right away as the seasons change helps you learn each plant's preferences intuitively over seasons spent together. Foundation herbs such as lavender, echinacea, and calendula offer a range of natural remedies and beauty, supplying your outdoor space and medicine cabinet. Accumulating familiarity with how these thrive and their functions allows them to become go-to companions in wellness. With patience and attentiveness, their generous support is repaid as trusted old friends.

Turning herbs into remedies requires extraction skills you now understand theoretically and soon practically. With various preparations, from tinctures to salves, you can craft powerful healing formulas. Safety, dosing, and interactions with medications require ongoing care and consultation with professionals. But you now have the core competencies to prepare high-quality herbal products for personal use.

While condensed here, these interconnected gardening and medicine-making skills could each fill their own book. Take your time to fully absorb each lesson by applying the knowledge. Start simply with a few herbs and tools before expanding the garden each year. Keep detailed notes on what works well in your unique environment. Prepare just one or two remedies in a season, slowly building knowledge of their uses and effects before adding more variety.

Above all, remember that herbalism is a lifelong journey. Growing medicinal plants connects you intimately to nature's healing abundance. Preparing your remedies instills self-reliance, creativity, and confidence. But always maintain a beginner's mind, approaching plants and people with humility and openness to new lessons.

Before rushing ahead to expand your garden, take time to care for and observe your starter herbs. Sit with a cup of tea among the plants at different times of the day. Through quiet contemplation, you may discover unexpected medicinal uses. Befriend herbs slowly to understand their unique personalities. Established plants, like lavender, become steady companions. The fast-growing calendula offers lessons in change and rebirth each season.

Making even one simple preparation, like calendula salve, teaches more than any book. Slowly craft it from start to finish, observing your materials and methods. Then patiently observe its effects on your skin compared to a store-bought product. You will intuitively learn so much more from purposeful, hands-on practice. Quality over quantity remains the best approach in herbalism.

Along the journey, remember that herbalism extends beyond growing plants and making formulas. Creating a community to share knowledge brings meaning and joy. Whether online or in person, surround yourself with people who inspire and challenge you. Consider joining our Facebook community, Herbs, Hearts, and Healing, and share not just your successes but also your failures, questions, and revelations. Avoid dogma or rigid rules, instead foster an open and supportive environment for everyone to learn and grow. Welcome diverse perspectives to expand your understanding. When you encounter contrary views, embrace the opportunity for respectful dialogue.

Nurture your health and well-being as diligently as any herb garden. Strengthen your body through good nutrition, regular exercise, and restful sleep. Feed your mind by setting aside time for reflection, creativity, and new challenges. Soothe your emotional spirit through practices like meditation, time in nature, journaling, or any activity that instills inner calm and purpose. Just as herbs thrive when their basic needs are met, you will blossom by tending to your holistic health.

Above all, maintain curiosity, patience, and gratitude along the journey. Let each herb and remedy teach you through direct experience. Give your full attention to every garden task and healing ritual. Express sincere appreciation to the plants, teachers, community, and living earth that sustain us. Herbalism is not just a skill but a way of life in kinship with nature. By infusing your practice with mindfulness and reverence, you allow herbal wisdom to transform you from the inside out. The rest unfolds gradually, each season building upon the last.

Herbalism will challenge and inspire you for a lifetime. But the fundamentals shared here equip you with all you need to begin. Start simply and nourish curiosity. The plants themselves will guide you, revealing their gifts slowly to those who care for them with an open and generous spirit. Trust in the process. You now have the tools and understanding to start growing healing herbs and making natural remedies that instill self-reliance, a deep connection with nature, and improved well-being. Be patient with yourself, celebrate small successes, and enjoy the journey ahead. If you've found this book to be helpful in any way, we ask that you please leave a simple review or rating on Amazon. Your support is greatly appreciated. Until next time and may your herbal pathways ever unwind with the seasons!

Thanks For Reading!

Hey! Thanks for taking the time to read this and may the seeds of knowledge we've planted grow and flourish. One last thing, and at this point we probably sound like a broken record, but it would mean a great deal to us if you left a review. Also, don't forget to grab your freebie if you haven't already! Just scan the code. See you in the Facebook group!

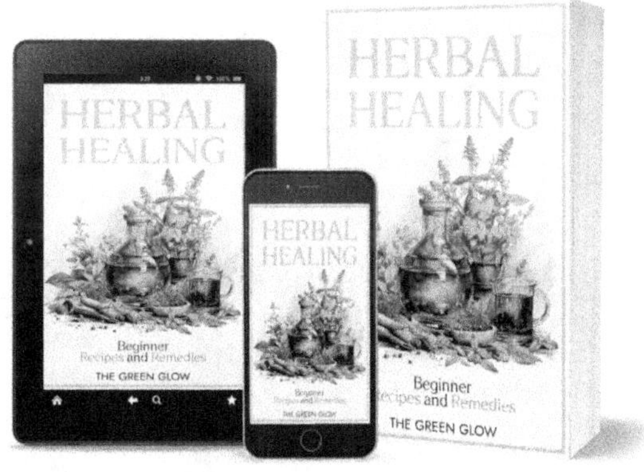

Yes, I almost forgot my freebie

Bibliography

12 essential herbs for your kitchen garden. (2022, June 20). Franks Nursery. https://franksnurseryandcrafts.com/12-essential-herbs-for-your-kitchen-garden/

Aziz, M. A., Khan, A. H., Adnan, M., & Ullah, H. (2018). Traditional uses of medicinal plants used by indigenous communities for veterinary practices at bajaur agency, pakistan. *Journal of Ethnobiology and Ethnomedicine, 14.* https://doi.org/10.1186/s13002-018-0212-0

Basicmedicalkey Admin. (2016, July 18). *Dosage and dosage forms in herbal medicine.* Basicmedical Key. https://basicmedicalkey.com/dosage-and-dosage-forms-in-herbal-medicine/

Better Health Channel. (2012). *Herbal medicine.* Better Health Channel. https://www.betterhealth.vic.gov.au/health/ConditionsAndTreatments/herbal-medicine

Building and maintaining a compost pile. (n.d.). Rutgers. Retrieved December 25, 2023, from http://www.rutgersln.com/nursery/gardening-info/building-and-maintaining-a-compost-pile/

Chapter 4, building and maintaining a compost pile. (n.d.). Aggie Horticulture. https://aggie-horticulture.tamu.edu/earthkind/landscape/dont-bag-it/chapter-4-building-and-maintaining-a-compost-pile/

Commission E: Browse monographs. (n.d.). American Botanical Council. Retrieved December 25, 2023, from http://cms.herbalgram.org/commissione/index.html?ts=1703507836&signature=6f27a4ebf73fea7b70ba2f5675d10ddc

CommonFloor Editorial Team. (2013, July 19). *Things to consider when choosing herbs for your garden.* CommonFloor. https://www.commonfloor.com/guide/things-to-consider-when-choosing-herbs-for-your-garden-26756

Davis, J. G., & Whiting, D. (n.d.). *Choosing a soil amendment.* Colorado State University. https://extension.colostate.edu/topic-areas/yard-garden/choosing-a-soil-amendment/

De Smet, P. A. (1995). Health risks of herbal remedies. *Drug Safety, 13*(2), 81–93. https://doi.org/10.2165/00002018-199513020-00003

Fields, D. (2016, August). *What is pharmacognosy?* News-Medical. https://www.news-medical.net/health/What-is-Pharmacognosy.aspx

Galor, S. W., & Benzie, I. F. F. (2011). *Herbal medicine.* Nih.gov. https://www.ncbi.nlm.nih.gov/books/NBK92773/

Hamidpour, M., Hamidpour, R., Hamidpour, S., & Shahlari, M. (2014).

Chemistry, pharmacology, and medicinal property of sage (salvia) to prevent and cure illnesses such as obesity, diabetes, depression, dementia, lupus, autism, heart disease, and cancer. *Journal of Traditional and Complementary Medicine*, 4(2), 82–88. https://doi.org/10.4103/2225-4110.130373

Hawk, M. (2022, February 7). *Dr. Elaine Ingham – the ecology of the soil food web*. Nature's Archive - a Podcast and More. http://naturesarchive.com/2022/02/07/soil/

Herbs at a glance. (n.d.). NCCIH. https://www.nccih.nih.gov/health/herbsataglance

Herman, A., Herman, A. P., Domagalska, B. W., & Młynarczyk, A. (2012). Essential oils and herbal extracts as antimicrobial agents in cosmetic emulsion. *Indian Journal of Microbiology*, 53(2), 232–237. https://doi.org/10.1007/s12088-012-0329-0

Housing news desk. (2023, March 16). *Herb garden: Facts, benefits, main plants, growing and caring tips.* Housing.com. https://housing.com/news/how-to-create-and-maintain-herb-gardens/

IARC Working Group on the Evaluation of Carcinogenic Risk to Humans. (2012). *Introduction.* Nih.gov; International Agency for Research on Cancer. https://www.ncbi.nlm.nih.gov/books/NBK326625/

Ioo, A. (2021, November 28). *What are the different types of soil amendments for your lawn?* Lawn Love. https://lawnlove.com/blog/different-types-of-soil-amendments/

Jauron, R., & Wallace, G. (2016, October 20). *Yard and garden: Constructing and managing compost piles.* Iowa State University. https://www.extension.iastate.edu/news/yard-and-garden-constructing-and-managing-compost-piles

Kaefer, C. M., & Milner, J. A. (2011). *Herbs and spices in cancer prevention and treatment.* Nih.gov; CRC Press/Taylor & Francis. https://www.ncbi.nlm.nih.gov/books/NBK92774/

Khalid, W., Arshad, M. S., Ranjha, M. M. A. N., Różańska, M. B., Irfan, S., Shafique, B., Rahim, M. A., Khalid, M. Z., Abdi, G., & Kowalczewski, P. Ł. (2022). Functional constituents of plant-based foods boost immunity against acute and chronic disorders. *Open Life Sciences*, 17(1), 1075–1093. https://doi.org/10.1515/biol-2022-0104

Lee, J. (2020, August 28). *Tincture making part 1: Macerations using dry herbs.* Homsted. https://www.homsted.com/blogs/homsted/tincture-making-101-macerations-using-dry-herbs/

Pan, S.-Y., Litscher, G., Gao, S.-H., Zhou, S.-F., Yu, Z.-L., Chen, H.-Q., Zhang, S.-F., Tang, M.-K., Sun, J.-N., & Ko, K.-M. (2014). Historical perspective of traditional indigenous medical practices: The current renaissance and conservation of herbal resources. *Evidence-Based Complementary and*

Alternative Medicine, 2014(525340), 1–20. https://doi.org/10.1155/2014/525340

Parham, S., Kharazi, A. Z., Bakhsheshi-Rad, H. R., Nur, H., Ismail, A. F., Sharif, S., RamaKrishna, S., & Berto, F. (2020). Antioxidant, antimicrobial and antiviral properties of herbal materials. *Antioxidants*, 9(12), 1309. https://doi.org/10.3390/antiox9121309

Petrovska, B. B. (2012). Historical review of medicinal plants' usage. *Pharmacognosy Reviews*, 6(11), 1. https://doi.org/10.4103/0973-7847.95849

Rahbardar, M., & Hosseinzadeh, H. (2020). Therapeutic effects of rosemary (Rosmarinus officinalis L.) and its active constituents on nervous system disorders. *Iranian Journal of Basic Medical Sciences*, 23(9). https://doi.org/10.22038/ijbms.2020.45269.10541

Sharma, A., Sabharwal, P., & Dada, R. (2021, January 1). *Chapter 1 - Herbal medicine—An introduction to its history* (R. Henkel & A. Agarwal, Eds.). ScienceDirect; Academic Press. https://www.sciencedirect.com/science/article/abs/pii/B9780128155653000011

Starting a medicinal garden. (2023, March 10). Zhi Herbals. https://www.zhiherbals.com/blog/guide-to-starting-a-medicinal-herb-garden

Stauffer, B., Carle, N., & Spuhler, D. (n.d.). *Soil amendment.* SSWM. https://sswm.info/water-nutrient-cycle/water-use/hardwares/conservation-soil-moisture/soil-amendment

Svedi, R. (2021, June 25). *Herb garden design - choosing a site for your herb garden.* Gardening Know How. https://www.gardeningknowhow.com/edible/herbs/hgen/choosing-a-site-for-your-herb-garden.htm

Vanderlinden, C. (2009). *The proper compost ratio of greens and browns.* The Spruce. https://www.thespruce.com/composting-greens-and-browns-2539485

Watts, S. (n.d.). *Herbal medicine - safe dosing and usage.* Mind Body Medical. Retrieved December 22, 2023, from https://www.mind-body-medical.co.uk/blog-weeklywisdom2/blog-post-title-one-bpxaf-rzetb-ncer8-7m92y-h3xwg-bly9x-7r4jn-cz7nb-fj8a4-sxg9f-x7wt3-xlbkw-fdgl2-46d9a-kkhxn-lxwmb-lzbbs-3s56w-clynh

WHO Team. (2000, November 12). *General guidelines for methodologies on research and evaluation of traditional medicine.* Www.who.int. https://www.who.int/publications/i/item/9789241506090

WishGarden Herbs. (2012, March 11). *General dosage guidelines for herbal tinctures.* WishGarden Herbs. https://www.wishgardenherbs.com/blogs/wishgarden/general-dosage-guidelines-for-herbal-tinctures-2

Yuan, H., Ma, Q., Ye, L., & Piao, G. (2016). The traditional medicine and modern medicine from natural products. *Molecules*, 21(5), 559. https://doi.org/10.3390/molecules21050559

Bibliography

Adaes, S. (2018, August 12). *Rhodiola rosea: medicinal use & science behind it.* Organic Boost. https://organicboost.com/rhodiola-rosea-medicinal-use/

American Botanical Council. (2023). *The ABC clinical guide.* Herbal gram. https://www.herbalgram.org/resources/abc-clinical-guide/

American Herbal Pharmacopoeia. (2023). American Herbal Pharmacopoeia. https://herbal-ahp.org/

American Herbal Products Association. (2022). Ahpa.org. https://www.ahpa.org/

American Herbalists Guild. (2013, June 2). *Herbal medicine faqs.* https://www.americanherbalistsguild.com/herbal-medicine-fundamentals

Badger, A. (2018, November 8). *3 ways to tap into an herbal community near you.* Urban Moonshine. https://www.urbanmoonshine.com/blogs/blog/3-ways-to-tap-into-an-herbal-community-near-you

Better Health Channel. (2021). *Herbal medicine.* https://www.betterhealth.vic.gov.au/health/conditionsandtreatments/herbal-medicine

Brinkley, E. (2022, October 10). *Optimizing social connection with herbs.* Dancing Willow Herbs. https://dancingwillowherbs.com/blogs/news/optimizing-social-connection-with-herbs

Canivenc-Lavier, M.-C. & Bennetau-Pelissero, C. (2023). Phytoestrogens and health effects. *Nutrients,* 15(2), 317-317. https://doi.org/10.3390/nu15020317

Cassie. (2020, March 11). *3 herbal recipes to enhance your intuition:* Zennedout. https://zennedout.com/3-herbal-recipes-to-enhance-your-intuition/

Champagne, É., Royo, A. A., Tremblay, J. & Raymond, P. (2019). Phytochemicals involved in plant resistance to leporids and cervids: a systematic review. *Journal of Chemical Ecology,* 46(1), 84–98. https://doi.org/10.1007/s10886-019-01130-z

Charlemagne. (n.d.). *Charlemagne quotes.* Quote Fancy. https://quotefancy.com/quote/1710220/Charlemagne-Herbs-are-the-friend-of-the-physician-and-the-pride-of-cooks

Chappell, S. (2019, February 21). *A beginner's guide to making herbal salves and lotions.* Healthline Media. https://www.healthline.com/health/diy-herbal-salves

Charles Sturt University. (2023). *Virtual herbarium.* Science Health CSU. https://science-health.csu.edu.au/herbarium

Corinne, J. (2021, June). *5 must have wellness teas to have in your pantry.* SKN Clinic. https://sknclinic.ca/2021/06/01/5-must-have-wellness-teas-to-have-in-your-pantry/

David Winston's Center for Herbal Studies. (2023). Herbal studies. https://herbalstudies.net/

DeJohn, S. (2023). *Herbs for health*. Garden. https://garden.org/learn/articles/view/2236/Herbs-for-Health/

Emerson, R. W. (n.d.). *Ralph Waldo Emerson quotes*. Fsm statistics. https://fsmstatistics.fm/plants-quotes/

Fletcher, J. (2019, January 10). *What is an herbal tincture? Recipes and uses*. Medical News Today. https://www.medicalnewstoday.com/articles/324149

World class botanical events and education for free! (2013). Free herbalism project. https://freeherbalismproject.com/

Gaia Herbs. (2021). Gaia Herbs. https://www.gaiaherbs.com/

Gladstar, R. (n.d.). *Rosemary Gladstar quotes*. Good reads. https://www.goodreads.com/search?utf8=%E2%9C%93&q=Rosemary+Gladstar&search_type=quotes

Gopal, S., Ajgaonkar, A., Kanchi, P., Kaundinya, A., Thakare, V., Chauhan, S., & Langade, D. (2021). Effect of an ashwagandha (Withania Somnifera) root extract on climacteric symptoms in women during perimenopause: A randomized, double-blind, placebo-controlled study. *Journal of Obstetrics and Gynaecology Research, 47*(12), 4414-4425.

Gregory, P. (n.d.). *Philippa Gregory quotes*. Good reads. https://www.goodreads.com/quotes/491242-in-a-way-magic-is-the-act-of-making-a

Griggs, B. (n.d.). *Barbara Griggs quotes*. Fsm statistics. https://fsmstatistics.fm/herbalist-quotes/

Güçlü-Üstündağ, Ö., & Mazza, G. (2023). *Saponins: properties, applications and processing*. Critical Reviews in Food Science and Nutrition. https://www.tandfonline.com/doi/abs/10.1080/10408390600698197

Healthline. (2017, October 30). *Homegrown herbal remedies*. Healthline Media. https://www.healthline.com/health/herbal-remedies-from-your-garden

Herbal Encyclopedia. (2010, December 30). *Cross reference scientific names of herbs with common names easily*. https://cloverleaffarmherbs.com/scientific-names/

Hippocrates. (2019, December 18). *Hippocrates quotes*. Wise owl quotes. https://wiseowlquotes.com/hippocrates/

Hoshaw, C. (2021, May 14). *Herbal medicine 101: how you can harness the power of healing herbs*. Healthline Media. https://www.healthline.com/health/herbal-medicine-101-harness-the-power-of-healing-herbs

Iannotti, M. (2022). *Types of mulch and why you should use them*. The Spruce. https://www.thespruce.com/what-is-mulch-1402413

Jekyll, G. (2023). *Gertrude Jekyll quotes*. Brainy Quote. https://www.brainyquote.com/quotes/gertrude_jekyll_310275

Jones, T. (2017, October 20). *10 healthy herbal teas you should try*. Healthline Media. https://www.healthline.com/nutrition/10-herbal-teas

Bibliography

Kolen, R. (2022). *5 tips for preserving homemade & natural body care products.* Mountain Rose Herbs. https://blog.mountainroseherbs.com/5-tips-preserv ing-handcrafted-natural-bodycare-products

Littefield, S. (2023). *Nutrition you can grow in your garden.* Garden. https:// garden.org/learn/articles/view/3856/Nutrition-You-Can-Grow-In-Your-Garden/

Matthew Wood Institute of Herbalism. (2023). https://www. matthewwoodinstituteofherbalism.com/

Moorhouse, D. (2018, June 30). *Ancient Egyptian medicine.* Schools History. https://schoolshistory.org.uk/topics/medicine-through-time/ancient-egypt ian-medicine/

Moss, W. (2023). *Starting plants from seed.* Garden. https://garden.org/learn/ articles/view/4433/Starting-Plants-From-Seed/

Mountain rose herbs. (2022). *How herbalism helps communities blossom.* https://blog.mountainroseherbs.com/herbalism-helps-communities

Najafian, Y., Hamedi, S. S., Farshchi, M. K., & Feyzabadi, Z. (2018). Plantago major in traditional Persian medicine and modern phytotherapy: a narrative review. *Electronic Physician, 10*(2), 6390-6399. https://doi.org/10. 19082/6390

National Center for Complementary and Integrative Health. (2023). *Herbs at a glance.* NCCIH. https://www.nccih.nih.gov/health/herbsataglance

National Gardening Association. (2023). Garden. https://garden.org/

Neveln, V. (2016). *15 easy-to-grow herbs that are perfect for beginners.* Better Homes & Gardens. https://www.bhg.com/gardening/vegetable/herbs/easy-to-grow-herbs/

NT Contributor. (2003, August 26). *Herbal remedies: integration into conventional medicine.* Nursing Times. https://www.nursingtimes.net/archive/ herbal-remedies-integration-into-conventional-medicine-26-08-2003/

Pan, S.-Y., Litscher, G., Gao, S.-H., Zhou, S.-F., Yu, Z.-L., Chen, H.-Q., Zhang, S.-F., Tang, M.-K., Sun, J.-N., & Ko, K.-M. (2014). Historical perspective of traditional indigenous medical practices: the current renaissance and conservation of herbal resources. *Evidence-Based Complementary and Alternative Medicine, 2014*(525340), 1-20. https://doi.org/10.1155/2014/ 525340

Pande, K. (2021, October 29). *Does intuition play a role in modern herbal practice?* Herbal Reality. https://www.herbalreality.com/herbalism/western-herbal-medicine/intuition-herbal-medicine-practice/

Paracelsus. (n.d.). *Paracelsus quotes.* Brainy Quote. https://www.brainyquote. com/quotes/paracelsus_138349

Porta, C. (2023). *Botanical medicines: foundations and practical applications.* Bakken Center for Spirituality & Healing. https://csh.umn.edu/academics/ for-credit-courses/csph-5423-botanical-medicines-foundations-and-practi cal-applications

Richter, C. (2023). *Growing herbs indoors*. Garden. https://garden.org/learn/articles/view/36/Growing-Herbs-Indoors/

Rodale Institute. (2021, January 20). *Free downloadable resources*. https://rodaleinstitute.org/education/resources/

Rosemary Gladstar's science & art of herbalism. (2016, April 13). The Science & Art of Herbalism. https://scienceandartofherbalism.com/

Santos, C. M. M., & Silva, A. M. S. (2020). The antioxidant activity of prenylflavonoids. *Molecules*, 25(3), 696. https://doi.org/10.3390/molecules25030696

Simple Loose Leaf Tea Company. (2020, March 17). *8 simple, homemade herbal tea recipes*. Simple Loose Leaf Tea Company. https://simplelooseleaf.com/blog/herbal-tea/herbal-tea-recipes/

Social impact. (2018). Gaia Herbs. https://www.gaiaherbs.com/pages/social-impact

Sowmya Andole, Thumma, G., Praveen Kumar Kusuma, Narender Boggula, Jainendra Kumar Battineni, Bakshi, V. & Kiran Gangarapu. (2023). Medicinal plants against SARS-CoV/Corona virus infections: ethnopharmacology, chemistry, clinical, and preclinical studies. *Springer EBooks*, 1-24. https://doi.org/10.1007/978-3-030-83350-3_15-1

Stafford Madeer, L. (2023). *The community supported herbal medicine movement*. Herbal gram. https://www.herbalgram.org/resources/herbalgram/issues/88/table-of-contents/hg88orgnews_commherbmed/

Sullivan, J. (2020, August 7). *A delicious summertime mocktail for immunity*. Wish Garden Herbs. https://www.wishgardenherbs.com/blogs/wishgarden/incorporating-herbs-into-your-daily-life

Ruskovska, T., Massaro, M., Maria Annunziata Carluccio, Arola-Arnal, A., Muguerza, B., Wim Vanden Berghe, Declerck, K., Calabriso, N., Combet, E., Gibney, E. R., Gomes, A., Gonthier, M.-È., Kistanova, E., Irèna Krga, Mena, P., Morand, C., Santos, C. N., Sonia de Pascual-Teresa, Rodriguez-Mateos, A., & Egeria Scoditti. (2020). Systematic bioinformatic analysis of nutrigenomic data of flavanols in cell models of cardiometabolic disease. *Food & Function*, 11(6), 5040-5064. https://doi.org/10.1039/d0fo00701c

TeaUSA. (2013). *Brewing tea*. https://www.teausa.com/14521/brewing-tea

The Botanical Society of America. (2023). CMS Botany. https://cms.botany.org/home.html

The Herb Guide. (2023). *Herbal tea*. https://www.the-herb-guide.com/herbal-tea.html

The history of herbal medicine. (2020). New Chapter. https://www.newchapter.com/wellness-blog/the-history-of-herbal-medicine/

United plant savers. (2022, September 23). https://unitedplantsavers.org/

Vasilis, E. (2023). *The power of herbs in building unity through community* gardens: growing together and connecting through nature's bounty. Coohom. https://www.coohom.com/article/the-power-of-herbs-in-building-unity-through-community-gardens

Wack, M. (2021, August 27). *Types of herbal tea and their benefits.* Artful Tea. https://artfultea.com/blogs/wellness/types-of-herbal-tea-and-their-benefits

Weed, S. (2023). *Herbal medicine: advice, articles, books, workshops, intensives, apprenticeship, correspondence courses.* Susun Weed. http://www.susunweed.com/

World Health Organization. (2019, November 25). *Traditional, complementary and integrative medicine.* https://www.who.int/health-topics/traditional-complementary-and-integrative-medicine#tab=tab_1

Yutang, L. (2023). *Lin Yutang* quotes. Good reads. https://www.goodreads.com/quotes/122552-there-is-something-in-the-nature-of-tea-that-leads

Zhang, L., Virgous, C., & Si, H. (2019). Synergistic anti-inflammatory effects and mechanisms of combined phytochemicals. *Journal of Nutritional Biochemistry, 69,* 19-30. https://doi.org/10.1016/j.jnutbio.2019.03.009